S0-EAP-430

Dedicated to <u>You</u>
♥ with Love ♥
from Paul Noddings

RESPONSIBLE RECOVERY

*My Opinions on Overcoming Addiction
after Getting into Recovery Myself and Many Years of
Running a Sober Home*

Paul Noddings

Copyright © 2020 Paul Noddings

This book or any portion thereof may not be reproduced or used in any manner whatsoever without the express written permission of the publisher except for the use of brief quotations in a book review.

Disclaimer

I am not a doctor. I do not offer any medical advice and I recommend the use of qualified doctors for medical advice. I am not a licensed therapist, psychologist, or drug counselor, and I recommend the use of these professionals. This is a book that details my opinions about recovery from addiction, after getting clean and sober myself and having gained a large amount of "boots-on-the-ground" experience running a sober home.

Acknowledgments

I would like to acknowledge Stefan J. Reich. Stefan came to Gault House as a client and then joined the management team. Stefan has been the House Manager of Gault House for several years. Stefan wrote the chapter entitled "Drugs Most Commonly Used, Illicit and Medically Assisted Treatment." I am very thankful to Stefan for his professional contribution to this book and to Gault House.

A Note to the Reader

There are case studies at the end of most chapters and several additional case studies at the end of this book. Some names have been altered to protect the privacy of those individuals. These case studies are interviews with addicts who have lived at the sober living home that I run. If you prefer to listen to these case studies, an audio version of them is available on the podcast page of our website.

These case studies are powerful and authentic. If they slow your progress to absorb the information in this book, skip them and come back to them at the end.

www . Responsible Recovery . net

Contents

Chapter 1: My Story

My name is Paul, and I am an alcoholic and a drug addict. Today, I am clean and sober, and I have been since January 6, 2015. I am also a landlord, who has years of experience running a residential complex in Santa Cruz, California, as a sober home.

I grew up on the coast of South Africa, and it was a good life. My parents were very loving and we went to the beach often. I loved to swim in the sea. By the age of 10, I had my own surfboard and I identified as a "surfer." Now I am much older (56 years old at the time of this writing), and I still surf and I still identify as a "surfer." Surfing is a healthy activity, an outdoors lifestyle. It is also a culture that has some dark spots. Heavy drug use was not common within my circle of surfing friends, though alcohol and marijuana was common. As a young surfer, I looked up to the older surfers. Most of them were drinking beer and hard liquor and smoking weed. As I got older and stronger and became a better surfer, I was included in the group of older boys, and soon I was drinking and smoking too.

This was innocent experimentation, in my opinion. It is normal development of a teenage boy into a young man. My problems came much further down the line. I continued surfing throughout college, and I continued drinking beer and smoking weed. I tried smoking cigarettes, but I didn't like them. They tasted foul to me; however, I liked smoking weed because it made me feel relaxed.

My habit" was to "have a few beers" and then a smoke of weed" and have a few more beers and another smoke of weed and then have a few more beers and another smoke of weed. After six beers and three joints (or bong hits), I was loaded and definitely over the limit to drive a vehicle. If a person does this once a month and stays at home while doing it, in my opinion, it is not a big problem. The problem for me is that I was doing this every night and I did this for 33 years, from age 18 to age 51. In addition, there was a progression in how much drinking and smoking I was doing.

I always worked hard, doing intellectually demanding work during the day, and after work, I would play hard by surfing, playing rugby, and hitting the gym, but at night, in order "to relax," I would smoke weed and drink beer. My problems with alcohol and marijuana were getting bigger, and I knew it for at least 10 years before I was able to stop. I tried to stop smoking weed many times, but it was never successful for more than a few days.

I was single, as I had never married, and I wanted to be with a loving partner. I had girlfriends over the years, but these relationships seemed to come to an abrupt end, and I would spend six months trying to figure out what went wrong before I would try again with someone new.

When I got loaded in the evenings, I would stay at home because I knew that I would not be able to attract anyone who I would be interested in when I was "bleeding from the eyes" and unable to talk without slurring my words. I found the loneliness crushing. On several occasions, I cried into my hands, because I was so lonely. It seemed that beer and weed were preventing me from finding a partner, but I was not able to stop using them and this seemed to be a vicious circle with no solution.

Then something dramatic happened. I went surfing at a surf break called "Four Mile." It is four miles north of Santa Cruz, California, where I had lived for 15 years. I had been surfing Four Mile as my main break for many years. On this day, I didn't walk along the base of the cliff to get into the water from the rocks, as I normally did, but rather I used the current to take me into the middle of the bay and I paddled toward the break. While I was in deep water in the middle of the bay, the dorsal fin of a large shark came to the surface of the water and it was swimming straight toward me at a fast speed. I was in a very bad position!

I was certain that this would be my last day alive. I thought that I would die in a pool of blood and bubbles and no-one would know until my surfboard washed up onto the beach. The shark was swimming straight at me, and I could see a fountain of water coming off each side of the dorsal fin. Time slowed down and my life flashed before me, including all the things that I had NOT done and that I had always thought that I would do, specifically getting married and having a child. My fear was extremely high, but I remained calm enough to make the decision to face the shark head-on and fight it. The shark submerged inches from the front of my surfboard and passed underneath me, and I turned, expecting it to come up behind me. It didn't, so

I started paddling as fast as I could to safety.

It took at least two minutes to get to safety and my adrenaline was so high that I was not able to sleep for 72 hours. I couldn't even lie down for more than a few minutes. I was so wide awake that I had to walk around the town of Santa Cruz through the middle of the night for two nights in a row. This scary event is still a major focal point for me, letting me know what is important to me. As my life flashed before me, smoking weed and drinking beer was not on my list of important things to do.

I was not able to stop smoking and drinking immediately after this scary event, but it was the catalyst that propelled me forward toward recovery and leading a full life. After I had become serious about recovery from addiction, I relapsed four or five times before I was successful in overcoming my addiction. With each relapse, I got a little smarter about what would cause the relapse and I got a little more understanding of my personal problems that manifest as addiction. I realized that for me "alcohol and weed" went together like "bacon and eggs." I knew that I had to stop BOTH to stop either.

A major asset to me in overcoming my addiction is Alcoholics Anonymous. I will forever be grateful to AA. The first time I went to an AA meeting near my home, introducing myself, "My name is Paul and I am an alcoholic and an addict," a huge weight was lifted off my shoulders. I had admitted to a room of peers that I had a problem, and the problem seemed to become more manageable as a result.

No one did anything especially for me or gave me specific advice that I remember. It was simply me admitting my problems to others and knowing there is a place to go where there are other people who openly admit they have problems that manifest as addiction that are too big for them to handle on their own. That was a major step forward for me. It has become more and more clear to me that this type of HONESTY is extremely important to recovery!

I planned my detox date and I struggled hard to not use drugs or alcohol for the first few days. I was constantly telling myself "NO!" The first week was very difficult and the first month was almost as difficult. After three months, I felt that I had too much to lose to relapse. After six months, I felt much more "in control" of myself. It was also around the six-month mark that I could feel myself moving toward "a new life," rather than constantly telling myself "NO" to my previous life.

I believe it took approximately two years for me to realize all the benefits of being clean and sober, specifically the mental clarity for which I am particularly thankful. Now I occasionally get cravings to use alcohol or marijuana, but they don't last long and thoughts of using are replaced with thoughts about the chaos and misery that drugs and alcohol will bring into my life.

Years after my scary event with the shark at Four Mile, I asked my girlfriend to handle the camera, while I stood in front of the camera, and we made a video entitled "Surfing with a Shark at Four Mile," which is on YouTube.

After shooting this video and with the camera still rolling, I knelt down on one knee and asked my girlfriend to marry me. At the time of writing this book, my wife and I have a very active son, who is already learning to surf!

I own a four-unit rental property, and as these units became available to rent to new tenants, I replaced the tenants with people who want to live in a sober living environment. I live on this property with my family, and we manage the property, along with a small management team who are clients. My years of "boots-on-the-ground" experience that I have gained from running this property, and my personal journey of recovery from addiction, are the basis of this book.

The recovery lifestyle is a much happier and healthier lifestyle than a life of alcohol and drugs. I am very pleased to be clean and sober, and I hope this book will help you in your struggle with addiction and your desire to be clean and sober yourself.

—Paul Noddings

Chapter 2: What Is Addiction?

Addiction always starts as casual use. There is ALWAYS a slide into addiction and it is a slippery slope.

Wikipedia defines addiction as a brain disorder characterized by compulsive engagement in rewarding stimuli despite adverse consequences. Google defines addiction as a psychological and physical inability to stop consuming a chemical, drug, activity, or substance, even though it is causing psychological and physical harm.

There is a big difference between "a party animal" and "an addict." Implied in the expression "party animal" is the concept that there is a party going on, and that would mean that there are other people around. If your life is all about parties, maybe you are an addict. If you attend one party per month and you really go wild, you are just a "a party animal."

There will be people who read this book who are consuming more alcohol or drugs than they would like, but who are not "full-blown addicts" like the case studies in this book. They may wish to reduce their consumption of drugs or alcohol, but not stopping completely. Reducing your consumption can be very difficult because once you have had one or two drinks (or lines of cocaine or any other drug), it is very difficult to not have a third or fourth.

All the recommendations in this book apply to people who want to reduce their consumption. If you are one of these people, I challenge you to stop consuming drugs or alcohol for 30 days. Your mind can play tricks on you and subconsciously come up with a really good reason why it is "okay" for you to break your commitment to not use drugs or alcohol for 30 days. If you cannot stop, perhaps you should acknowledge that you have an addiction? Perhaps you should stop using drugs and alcohol permanently before you do more harm to yourself and others around you. A sober life is more fun and more meaningful than a life of substance abuse and there are many benefits of being clean and sober.

More people are addicted to alcohol than any other drug! Many of them are in denial. The reason, in part, is that alcohol is accepted within our society, as it is commonly available and often encouraged.

Alcohol can cause death by seizure, but it causes one-hundred-fold more problems, such as road accidents, injury to people doing something stupid that they would not do while sober, physical fights, and relationship problems, the break-up of marriages, mood swings, hangovers, poor judgment, incorrect conclusions, indifference to the consequence of actions, and many other problems.

Here are a few questions to help you to know if you have a problem with alcohol:

- Do you have three or more DUIs (driving under the influence)?
- Do you go to a different bar each night of the week so that the barman does not see you too often?
- Do you have a favorite bar where everyone knows your first name?

- Do you buy large bottles of hard alcohol because it is cheaper by volume?
- Do you drink alcohol every night?
- Do you drink alcohol shortly after waking up?
- Do you need to drink alcohol in order to go to sleep?

I have traveled to many countries and it seems that in every country there are many people who are drinking alcohol or getting loaded with whatever is available. Even in the jungles of the Amazon, Indian tribes have special potions to "get off their head." Humans seem to have a need (or at least a strong desire) to get wasted. In my opinion, this will not change and it is not my intention to change it. Many people can use drugs or alcohol occasionally and it is my hope that they can do so safely for themselves and others.

My goal is to assist people who started off using drugs or alcohol occasionally and then found themselves using drugs and alcohol more and more often, and then "suddenly," they have an addiction problem they don't know how to solve.

Most addicts go through a period of denial where they try to convince themselves and others around them that they do not have an addiction problem. Ninety-nine percent of addicts will "hit rock bottom" and be forced to confront their problems, and they will eventually "know within their heart" that they have an addiction problem.

This book focuses on addiction to drugs and alcohol. Most of the lessons in this book can be adapted to help people who are addicted to sex, food, gambling, social media, TV, gaming, relationships, a need to be liked, etc.

To fix a problem of addiction, it is essential that the ADDICT acknowledges that there is "a problem." This acknowledgement is critical. The addict has to take responsibility for fixing their problem of addiction. No one else can do it for them.

Below is a list of some characteristics of addiction. These questions will give you an idea of where you are on the spectrum of addiction:

- Do you get loaded while alone?
- Do you get loaded regularly, like every day?
- Do you get loaded seven days a week?
- Do you get loaded shortly after waking up?
- Do you get loaded more than once a day?
- Do you get loaded even though you don't want to get loaded?
- Do you promise yourself that you will stop getting loaded but find that you continue to get loaded?
- Do you feel that your world is closing in on you?
- Do you feel that your world is getting smaller and smaller?
- Have you had blackouts in your memory due to substance abuse?
- Do you get absolutely hammered on a regular basis?
- Do you lose jobs due to substance abuse?
- Do you steal in order to sell the stolen items to get money for drugs or alcohol?
- Do you lie repeatedly to cover up your drug and alcohol use?
- Have you been arrested multiple times for drug or alcohol offenses?
- Have you been told by multiple people that you have a drug or alcohol problem?

- Does it leave you sick if you do NOT use drugs or alcohol?
- Do you feel very lonely while loaded?
- Do you feel that there is much missing from your life while loaded?
- Do you feel trapped while loaded?

If you have answered yes to many of these questions, the next step is to answer the question, "Do you want to fix this problem?"

If there is not a strong desire to fix the problem BY THE PERSON WHO HAS THE PROBLEM, there will not be much progress made in fixing the problem.

Wives, mothers, fathers, lovers, etc., begging, threatening, or beating an addict will not work; it is misdirected energy, even if it is well-intended.

It is the addict who MUST be the one who wants to recover from the addiction because it is the addict who must put in the effort to recover from this disease!

Chapter 3: Take Action Now

The path to recovery from addiction is NOT a secret. I have listed steps below that will help you. These steps are physical action steps. You do these steps with your actions. You don't need to over-think these steps; just do them. Following these steps does not guarantee you anything, but they make the chances of your success greater.

These steps are placed in order of priority, and I recommend that you follow them closely for at least six months:

1. Take Action: Stop Using and Detoxify
2. Take Action: Live with Other Sober People
3. Take Action: Get Healthy, Physically and Spiritually
4. Take Action: Keep a Diary
5. Take Action: Get Out and About
6. Take Action: Go to Recovery Meetings
7. Take Action: Get a Sponsor (or Two)
8. Take Action: Develop Your Own Program of Recovery
9. Take Action: Get a Job; it Provides Structure
10. Take Action: Contribute to Society and Help Others

If you are an addict and you want to stop using, you must be very serious about wanting to overcome your addiction! If you think that your problem is "not a problem," you are "stopping for someone else," or "your personal identity is created by your using," you will relapse quickly and your situation could be worse than before.

During the first six-month period, live ONE DAY AT A TIME! Do NOT over-think your situation; just follow these steps diligently and live "ONE DAY AT A TIME" until you have at least six months of clean time, and then you can assess your situation again.

In early recovery, most addicts will think about using every day, often multiple times every day. Do NOT use! Try to live moment to moment until your cravings pass. To quiet your mind, ask yourself the question, "Are my thoughts useful and how do they behave?"

Change happens when you feel pain. Embrace the pain, but do not surrender to it. Channel the energy toward achieving your goal of getting clean and staying sober.

1. Take Action: Stop Using and Detoxify

If you are an addict and you want to stop your addiction, you MUST stop using. For most people, going "cold turkey" is NOT a good idea. There are many addiction treatment centers that specialize in detoxing addicts. I recommend that you use these facilities.

Most detox centers cost approximately $1,000 per day and are run similar to a hospital, and most will require a minimum of a one-week stay. Many health insurance providers will cover some or all of these costs. If this route is above your financial means, you MUST look for an opening within a county detox program.

I understand that many counties do not have enough beds or money to fund these detox programs, meaning that an addict with little funds has to stay addicted until an opening is available.

I have heard of people renting a room in a house for a week for the specific purpose of getting off the streets and trying to stay clean for a week. This is dangerous and not what I recommend. I recommend showing your seriousness about recovery by camping on the doorstep of the detox center and other nonviolent methods of communication to show how serious you are about overcoming addiction.

I believe that if you are truly serious about recovery, you will find an opening in a detox program somewhere, and when you get your chance, you must take it with both hands.

When I stopped using, it was difficult. I had to tell myself "No" many times every day, especially the first few weeks. I found the tools listed below very helpful to get me through the first days and then weeks and months. Try them and if you fail, don't give up, learn from your failure and try again!

2. Take Action: Live with Other Sober People

In my opinion, it is absolutely ESSENTIAL that immediately after detox, you live with other people who are clean and sober, for example, in a well-run sober home. The camaraderie and support that you can get from other people in a sober home, who have traveled the same path that you are on, is very valuable to your success.

Do NOT return to the living environment that you were in during your using days, whether that was your parents' house, your house, your car, a place you shared with "friends," or the streets.

Sober homes are structured living environments where you agree to abide by the structure, and if you fail to abide by the structure, you agree to leave the home immediately. The people that run sober homes are NOT your parents and they are NOT going to beg you to abide by the structure. If you don't follow the structure, you will be given a warning or two and then be asked to leave so that the home can function as it is intended to function, which is as a well-run sober home for people who are serious about overcoming their addiction. Don't expect the sober home or the people who run the sober home to do the hard work for you. You are responsible for your own recovery.

Simply living with other people who are NOT using any drugs or alcohol themselves will help you to not use drugs or alcohol yourself. Part of the reason to live in a sober home is the positive influence from the other people who are living there and from the structure of the home, but another good reason to live in a sober home is to NOT be living where you were when you were using. The people who were around you during your using period need to be replaced with new people who are NOT using drugs or alcohol. This means getting rid of old "friends" and it can also mean redefining your relationship with family members who may be using drugs or alcohol.

3. Take Action: Improve Your Health, Physically and Spiritually

These subjects need to be broken down into several topics, and each of these topics has been the sole subject of many books and YouTube channels. Here I am concerned with the basics of good health, breaking this big subject down into the following subtopics:

A. Sleep
B. Food
C. Exercise
D. Stop Smoking
E. Spiritual Health

A. Sleep

Sleep and adequate rest is appropriate for people who are overcoming addiction, but NOT lying around all day doing nothing! Eight hours of sleep is enough and if you need 10 hours, go ahead. That still leaves 14 hours, during which time you should be awake, dressed, bed made, and doing something productive. Going to bed a few hours after the sun has gone down is recommended.

If you are in recovery, do NOT do night work (graveyard shift), as it will reduce your chances of success. Get your daily sleep cycle coordinated with the daily cycle of the earth and the sun. This may sound cliché but it is important that you get your sleep cycle "in harmony with the universe."

Most sleep experts recommend a consistent routine around sleep, such as going to bed at the same time each night, turning off mental stimulants such as lights and screen time at least one hour before bedtime, calming your mind, making your sleep area comfortable and attractive, and not consuming a stimulant like coffee at least four hours before your bedtime.

Good sleep is important to good health. Putting effort into getting good sleep is worth your time.

B. Food

You may be surprised to see diet advice in a book on recovery from addiction, but I recommend removing all processed foods and all simple carbohydrates from your diet.

No simple carbohydrates means no sugar, candy, soda, ice cream, sweet fruit, pasta, rice, bread, potatoes, biscuits, etc. These simple carbohydrates are processed as glucose by the body. The glucose is quickly absorbed and stored, leaving you hungry again.

Your brain is mostly made of fat. Eating a high-fat diet appears to support brain function. About 40 percent of our clients are on the Keto diet and our clients have come to us from many different sources. It is surprising how many people who are all in recovery from addiction have independently decided to use the Keto diet. The calorie marcos of the Keto diet are 70 percent fat, 20 percent protein, and 10 percent carbohydrates, in the form of leafy green vegetables.

I recommend my personal combination of foods, which I call the "oily vegetable" diet. I recommend that your plate of food be prepared at home and that 80 percent of the plate be covered with plant-based, naturally grown salads and vegetables, with plenty of good oils such as olive oil, avocado oil, coconut oil, and butter from grass-fed cows. The remaining 20 percent of the surface area of your plate should be fatty and natural.

The saturated fat (meat) that I recommend is pork-belly. Bacon is thin-cut pork-belly. I prefer pork-belly over bacon because the bacon can have all the fat cooked out of it and I want the fat. Pork-belly is mostly fat (white in color) and not protein (red in color) and it is the fat that is helpful. Other fatty meat (cocked at a low temperature in coconut oil) include wild salmon for its omega-3 fatty acids, cuts of beef and lamb with plenty of white fat visible within the meat, and ground meat with a high fat content.

Ideally, your body will switch to burning fat for fuel rather than glucose. When this happens, your body can draw down on the energy stored in your fat cells. You may lose some excess body fat and you have longer periods without feeling hungry.

The brain is made up of fat mostly and I believe that your brain prefers its fuel source to be fat and your mood improves if your fuel source is mostly fat. When people are feeling good, they normally look good too.

I also recommend only two meals a day, brunch (10 a.m.) and dinner (4 p.m.), with no snaking between meals. This meal plan gives an "intermittent fasting period" of about 18 hours. It takes about 16 hours for your liver to put all the glucose it is able to store into your bloodstream, which should give you two hours of fat burning per day. If two meals a day are not enough for you, do three meals a day, with no snacking in between. It is important to stop snaking because it is an eating pattern of constant "grazing." The grazing food tends to be simple carbohydrates with loads of preservatives and sugar, in a plastic wrapper, with misleading marketing messages, such as "Health Bar". This is not good food for your brain and it does not support your recovery from addiction.

The beginning of your digestive tract is your mouth. Many people in recovery have neglected their dental hygiene and their teeth are in poor condition. Perhaps you can set a goal of getting your dental work done if you can stay off drugs and alcohol for one year, then spend some money on yourself and start the process of improving your teeth. You will look better and you will be able to eat better too.

C. Exercise

I believe that GENTLE exercise is good for everyone. Walking is possibly the best exercise of all. It is free and easy to do. You don't need to hike up the side of a mountain; just walk around your neighborhood regularly. Walk regularly throughout the day. Other gentle exercise options are swimming (slowly) and yoga and stretching. Yoga involves breathing and connecting to your body, which can calm your mind too.

I do not recommend heavy hardcore exercise until your recovery is solid. The stress on your body and the endorphins that are released may be a trigger for you to start using again.

I also do not recommend high-adrenaline activities. No parachuting, base-jumping, or wing-suit flights in early recovery! There are many other high-adrenaline activities and they do not go well with recovery. You will do better keeping yourself calm and doing light exercise. Exercise such as walking, bike riding, swimming, press-ups, sit-ups, and squats, all done at a low intensity, on a regular basis, will support your recovery.

D. Stop Smoking

In my opinion, about 70 percent of people in recovery are either smoking cigarettes or using a vaporizer. Both of these are unhealthy! There is no doubt that smoking is bad for your health. Quit smoking! If it is too much for you to quit smoking while quitting drugs and alcohol, come up with a plan to quit smoking at some point in time. Don't fool yourself; smoking is not good for your health. You should have a plan to remove this harmful activity from your life.

E. Spiritual Health

Meditation can be helpful to calm your mind and connect you to your spiritual self. You do not have to go to a class to meditate; just find a quiet place and go inside your mind. It can become easy if you practice it. The Buddhist concept of mindfulness is a good place to start if you want to look for help on this subject.

None of us choose to be born and we are all going to die. There are approximately 7 billion people on planet earth, a small number you care about and most you don't even know.

This huge collective consciousness is my "higher power." I try to orientate my personal psyche with my "higher power" to achieve spiritual peace.

Feeling spiritually centered allows you to handle your day-to-day struggles with more grace and well-being. Silent observation can assist you to dissolve your ego and become "one with the universe." Spiritual health promotes mental health and I encourage both.

4. Take Action: Keep a Diary

Keeping a diary is a big "bang-for-your-buck" tool that you can use to help you to overcome addiction! It is an easy tool for you to use and it will help you to get good results.

Keeping a diary is having a written conversation with yourself. The act of writing down thoughts is very helpful in straightening out your thoughts. As an added bonus, you get a written record of your thoughts. In my experience, I seldom review my diary entries. It is mostly the act of writing in my diary that is helpful because it forces me to organize my thoughts.

Keeping a diary can be the "old-fashioned" notebook and pen. If you are going this route, I recommend visiting a stationery store. For less than $10, you can get a small leather-bound notebook that will fit into the top pocket of a shirt. This way, the diary is easy to keep with you throughout the day.

A more modern alternative is to use your cell phone as a diary. Find an App that you like and use it to keep notes throughout the day.

For an addict in recovery, keeping written notes about your cravings and how you overcame those cravings can be very helpful in controlling yourself and getting though the early days.

Don't substitute talking to other people with keeping a diary. There is a difference between having a written conversation with yourself and having a conversation with another person.

5. Take Action: Get Out and About

Do NOT isolate. Most addicts will "isolate and medicate." Part of the definition of an addict is using drugs and alcohol while alone. It is unwise to do things that result in your prolonged isolation from other people. Some people will isolate while in a crowd. They will blend into the background, sit in the corner, and be depressed. Do NOT let this happen to you. Get involved with activities that keep your interest. Get out and about.

Some job functions are isolating by the nature of the job. Computer programming can cause the programmer to have little interaction with other humans and have their head inside a computer all day. You may have worked in a career job that has isolated you from people and society for years. If you are in recovery from addiction, that career may need to come to an end. Most people have four or five "career" jobs in their working lifetime. It is unrealistic to expect to do the same job for more than 10 years and a change can be refreshing. If you are in recovery from addiction and your job leaves you feeling isolated from people, find a new job ASAP. I recommend starting with entry- level jobs. These are easier to get and give you the opportunity to move up over time.

Working the graveyard shift is NOT recommended for people in recovery. Night work isolates people from the majority of society and there is evidence that correlates addiction with night work. Addicts should get their daily rhythm in line with the sun and the earth and get regular exposure to other regular people living a regular life.

6. Take Action: Go to Recovery Meetings

I highly recommend that recovery meetings be a major part of your personal recovery program, especially in early recovery. Many people do 90 meetings in 90 days. This is an excellent start. It gives you hope to see so many other people struggling with the same problems as you. It makes you realize that you are not alone. You are likely to make friends with some of the people at these meetings and these new friends can offer you support to stay clean as they are trying to do the same thing themselves.

After you have six months of clean time, you may scale back on your meeting attendance, but please do NOT stop going to meetings altogether because it is a common precursor to a relapse back to using drugs or alcohol. Many times I have heard people talk about how their meeting attendance reduced in the lead-up to their relapse.

I found AA meetings to be the most helpful for me. I have also attended NA meetings, Smart Recovery meetings,

Buddha Recovery meetings, and Al-anon meetings. I found Al-anon meetings VERY helpful too.

Do NOT sit at the back and say nothing. Participate in the meeting. Let other people get the meeting going and then contribute to the meeting with your input, whatever that may be. People who are new to recovery add to the quality of the meeting. You add fresh insight and help the other folks to keep up their efforts in recovery. Everyone is helping each other, so please contribute with your input.

7. Take Action: Get a Sponsor (or Two)

Recovery meetings are the best place to meet people who you can ask to be your sponsor. A sponsor is a "big brother" or "big sister" who will support you in your recovery journey. Sponsors are a common part of the AA recovery method and they will assist you to "work the 12 Steps." I did the 12 Steps, but I did not find them particularly helpful; however, I did find having sponsors very helpful and the concept of sponsors is not only related to the AA recovery method.

A sponsor is a mentor. They will talk to you about the journey of recovery that you are on. They will offer advice and they should be available for you to call them if you need to speak to someone urgently, particularly if you are having cravings to use drugs. Your sponsor should be able to talk you down from these cravings.

You should look for a sponsor who has many years of sobriety under their belt and they are solid in the sobriety. You should like this person and this person must have time for you. Some sponsors are popular and have multiple people that they are sponsoring, which can mean that they don't have much time for you.

In my opinion, it is a good idea to have more than one sponsor. One sponsor may be good at certain aspects of recovery but not others. Sponsors also change from time to time. You may get along well at first, but not so good later. Don't get frustrated with your sponsor. People who are willing to sponsor/mentor you are doing so because they are good people and you should aspire to sponsoring other people in your future.

I have several strong mentors with whom I am in daily contact (often hourly contact) and I find this VERY helpful. I recommend that everyone get a sponsor (or two or three) with whom you have daily contact and with whom you discuss all important decisions. A sponsor can be a great asset in making decisions.

8. Take Action: Develop Your Own Program of Recovery

I am a big supporter of AA (Alcoholics Anonymous) and NA (Narcotics Anonymous) and Al-Anon (support for the people who want to help an addict). AA recommends the 12-Step program, and there is a religious background to the teachings of AA. I am not a religious person; however, I am a spiritual person and I find it easy to use the "collective consciousness of humanity" as a substitute for the "higher power" to which AA refers frequently. In my personal recovery, I did not find the 12 Steps particularly helpful, even though I did work through them, and I recommend that everyone try the 12-Step program and that everyone use AA and their teachings, until you find a better recovery program more suited to you.

There are many other recovery programs available, including Intensive Out-Patient (IOP) programs, SMART Recovery, Buddha Recovery, Conscious Recovery, Spiritual Recovery, and Religious Recovery. I encourage you to try all of these programs and see which works best for you. It is not the case that "one size fits all."

Until you have found a better path for yourself, I highly recommend participating in AA or NA meetings regularly, finding a sponsor, and being very honest with yourself and everyone around you. Then develop your own program of recovery. Make it fit your life but have a serious program, one that you can write down and review this program with your sponsors so that you can be confident in your own program of recovery.

9. Take Action: Get a Job; it Provides Structure

In my opinion, getting a paid job is extremely important. A paid job is important for the structure that it brings to your life even more than the money it provides. A paid job is NOT attending college or doing volunteer work. The type of paid job that I am referring to is not working for yourself or your father, uncle, or some other relative who offers you protected employment. A paid job is when you have regular work hours and a defined set of tasks that you are expected to perform for an organization that is not treating you any differently

40

than it treats their other employees. (I also recommend that you inform your employer that you are in recovery from addiction, except if you "know for a fact" that it will have an adverse result on your position in the company.)

This structure is helpful to someone in recovery and it gives people a daily routine. At the early stages of recovery, it is most important that the recovering addict get out of the sober house, go to work, and get stimulus into their life from people other than just those people with whom they live in the sober home.

People who are early in recovery should NOT be looking for their dream job; an entry-level job or minimum-wage job is a better starting point. From this entry-level position, growth is likely. If you get a minimum-wage job, you increase the interest that another employer may have in employing you in a more senior position because you are demonstrating that you are capable of working by having the first job. There is no better position to find a good job than to have a job already. There is not an expectation that you be "super-loyal" to your minimum-wage job. If you change your minimum-wage job several times over a few months, it will not reflect poorly on you.

This is a good time to try a few different working environments. Outdoor work, such as tree cutting, construction, or delivery driver, may suit you, or indoor work, such as computer work, accounting, or office administration may be a good fit for you. The idea is to get any job to start with and then get a slightly better job doing things that you feel are a better fit for you. Then start building a plan for your longer-term goals.

10. Take Action: Contribute to Society, Be of Service and Help Others

Contributing to society will make you feel good about yourself! If you are feeling depressed; help other people, and you are more likely to feel happy. There is no better way to feel good about yourself than to help someone else. If you help someone who is obviously less fortunate than yourself, such as keeping company with a person who is confined to a bed, you are more likely to count your blessings. There are many opportunities to help other people. You don't need to join an organization to help others. Just go down to your local grocery store and talk to elderly people; most of them are lonely and would appreciate being noticed. Talking to people who don't get much attention from the rest of society is helpful to those people. Walk around and look for elderly, homeless, disabled, and poor people and talk to them nicely; it will help you feel better about your own situation.

One of the easiest ways "to be of service" is to help out at the AA or NA meetings or do more chores at your sober living home. After doing some immediate things to be of service and help others, you can join organizations that are set up to help others. There are food banks that need volunteers, kitchens feeding the homeless, sports events for disabled people, etc. You may meet new friends at these events.

I have noticed that people LOVE to watch someone else working. I have done plenty of property work, carpentry, plumbing, electrical, and landscaping, and people always find a reason to hang around and watch me work. At first, I did not like to be watched and I would tell people to "go away," as politely as I could, until I realized that people just love to watch other people doing work.

If it does not cause you stress and you can tolerate other people watching you while you work, you will become popular if you do loads of work and let people watch you do it. Being popular can be helpful for many people; it can make you feel good about yourself and it does not have the same risks as being in a serious relationship.

Many people want to be popular and they use social media or contort their personality to achieve it. I have found a simple way to be popular is to do work and allow people to watch you do it. It does not really matter what the work is; if people can watch you do it, they will like you.

If you contribute to society, are of service, and help others, you will be liked by other people and that will help you to feel good about yourself and stay on track with your recovery from addiction.

Chapter 4: Please Do NOT Do Any of These

Please do not do any of the actions or thoughts listed below. By not doing them, you significantly increase your chances of having a life free from drugs and alcohol.

The first two items listed below are "Do NOT Take Action" steps. These are actions that I ask that you do NOT do:

1. Do NOT go to people or places where drugs and alcohol are used
2. Do NOT get into a serious relationship

The last three items listed are "Control Your Mind" considerations that you should NOT do.

3. Do NOT let your guard down on alcohol
4. Do NOT convince yourself that you can do "a little" drugs or alcohol
5. Do NOT stress

1. Do NOT Take Action: Do NOT Go to People or Places Where Drugs and Alcohol Are Used

Everyone has heard the saying, "If you hang around a barbershop, soon you will have a haircut." Similarly, if you go to bars, soon you will be having a drink. For many addicts, all the people they know are using drugs and alcohol, so in order to overcome your addiction, you will need an entirely new set of friends. Do not hang out with people who you know are using drugs or alcohol. This includes family and good friends.

Start by making friends at AA meetings, recovery events, and the places where you are being of service. Know in advance you MUST make a new set of friends who do not use drugs or alcohol.

There can be very difficult situations within family settings where one or all of the family are using. Try to avoid these events until you are solid in your recovery. If you go to places or events where drugs are regularly consumed, it is likely that you will consume these drugs too. We all know that there is Ecstasy at raves, cocaine at night clubs, and meth at brothels. Don't go to these places.

If you have a year or more of sobriety and you "HAVE TO GO" to a bar, be prepared before you go. Tell the people you are going with about your situation. Order a bottle of water, sparkling if they have it. A bottle of cold water is surprisingly similar to a bottle of cold beer, except the drug "alcohol" is not included.

If you are new to recovery, do NOT go to people or places where drugs or alcohol are consumed!

2. Do NOT Take Action: Do NOT Get into Sexual Relationships

Sexual relationships are serious relationships and serious relationships are bad for people who are in early recovery, at minimum, the first six months of recovery from addiction, even if the other person is in recovery themselves.

Most sexual relationships fall apart at some point and this breakdown usually causes both people heartache, anger, anxiety, frustration, and stress. These emotions may send you running back to your drug of choice. Relationships are a major stress point for most people and can cause a relapse more than anything else.

Codependent relationships are some of the most toxic of all relationships. Among the core characteristics of codependency is an excessive reliance on the other person in the relationship for a sense of identity and approval. Many professionals within the field of addiction believe that an addict's relationship with their drug of choice is a codependent relationship.

Light, casual relationships are encouraged and these relationships are completely different from serious or sexual relationships because they do not cause stress in the same way that sexual relationships do. Professional relationships, with social workers or drug counselors, are also encouraged, and these relationships should cause no stress at all.

Humans are social animals: very few people "thrive" in isolation. Some people can tolerate isolation, but most people seek relationships. These relationships should be light and casual, friendly and positive, not sexual and not serious relationships, and definitely not codependent relationships.

Take an honest look at your relationships, with your parents, siblings, friends, and past lovers. It is a good idea to make a written list of all the relationships that you have had and write down information about the positives and negatives of each relationship. There is an old saying, "Show me your friends and I will know who you are." Write down the good and the bad of past relationships and you will learn the patterns that you follow.

There are many examples of very clever people getting married and then getting divorced. Being intelligent is not a prerequisite to having successful relationships. In my opinion, being "HUMBLE" is the best solution for lasting meaningful relationships. Being your own person, while allowing your partner in your relationship to "win most of the time" is what I mean by being "humble." Let them make the funniest joke or be the decider on which restaurant you eat at. Being humble also means allowing your partner to make major decisions as well as minor ones. It means giving up control and being comfortable as the "passenger on the bus" and not the "driver of the bus." Being humble can be difficult. It can cause you to feel frustrated and even angry.

As a person in recovery from addiction, it is important that you take responsibility for your life to get out of addiction, so this is not a good time to be humble and put control in the hands of a partner. A person who is in recovery from addiction is fighting for his or her life. This is NOT a good time to be building a life with another person.

Take control of your own life and be responsible for your own life. Leave serious relationships with other people out of your life until you have full control of your life and then be very careful with who you allow into your life.

Relationships with parents and siblings can be very complicated and these relationships are also very important.

As kids, and then teenagers, and then adults, we go through different stages in our relationships with parents. When we are adults ourselves, we are still highly influenced by our relationships with our parents. I recommend professional help if you have problems in this area.

It is unrealistic for someone to succeed in recovery while having a sexual relationship with someone who is actively using drugs or alcohol. A couple may be drinking together or shooting heroin together. If one person wants to get clean and the other doesn't, the person wanting to get clean will have to LEAVE the other person and their relationship. People who are deep in addiction are fighting for their life. You have a better chance if you are on your own.

In our sober homes, couples are not accepted, and if a sexual relationship develops, both people have to leave. There are many opportunities for men and woman living in a sober home to "hook up." This will decrease the chances of successful recovery for both individuals. I have seen many examples of clients developing a sexual relationship, moving out of sober living to be with that person, and then relapsing.

I do NOT recommend sexual relationships for anyone in early recovery!

3. Control Your Mind: Do NOT Let Your Guard Down on Alcohol

Alcohol has been "grandfathered" into our society as if it was different from other drugs, but it is NOT. It is a mood-altering, brain-fogging, endorphin-releasing chemical high like all the other drugs.

Way back in the 1920s, there was a period of "Prohibition" when alcohol was outlawed. Similar to the "War on Drugs," Prohibition failed. Alcohol manufacture and distribution went underground, into the hands of criminals, proliferating in society more than ever.

Now alcohol consumption is widely accepted within society, even encouraged. Sportsmen and women, firefighters and police, office workers and colleagues, are expected to enjoy "a few drinks" after work. Children see adults consuming alcohol from an early age and this attracts children to try it. Alcohol is one of the most commonly available drugs. Grocery stores sell it, convenience stores sell it, and it is advertised in the movies and on TV.

In my opinion, alcohol is the worse drug of all and it is the primary gateway drug to other drugs. Almost every addict who I have interviewed has told me that they started off by using alcohol. I believe that alcohol caused more deaths, directly and indirectly, than any other drug and that it makes people aggressive and not care about the consequences of their actions.

Even if your drug of choice is not alcohol, you are more likely to use your drug of choice after you have "had a few drinks."

In the sober home that I run, at least 40 percent of my clients are here to recover from alcohol as their primary drug of choice. I had a client leave our sober home and then die from alcohol and alcohol was the direct cause of a long-term incarceration of another client who deliberately rammed a police car while driving drunk. In addition to these two examples, alcohol has caused multiple relapses and the eviction of multiple clients.

The client who was incarcerated for deliberately ramming a police car was approximately one month into his sobriety when he decided to watch a football match at a "sports bar." Soon he was drinking "a few beers" with a "friend"; then he was snorting cocaine with his "friend." He got hammered and he decided to drive home. When a police car lit up its lights behind him, he spun his car around and rammed into the police car. The Police Department and the District Attorney take these things very seriously and this person got 10 years in jail. It all started with "a few beers."

The most expensive advertising slots on U.S. television are at the halftime break of the NFL Super Bowl event and most of these advertisers are beer companies. These beer companies want to sell the message, "Enjoy a few cold beers," but the reality is that very few people can limit their consumption to "just a few cold beers."

Most people get "buzzed" on beer and then switch to harder alcohol to get drunk. Many people will use cocaine or other speed products so that they can drink more alcohol and get really hammered.

A person with an addiction to meth or heroin has very little chance to say "no" to meth or heroin once they are "buzzed."

In my opinion, all alcohol purchases should be recorded in a computerized database. Every purchase of alcohol should be recorded so that it is clear what qualities of alcohol a particular person is consuming. This would allow services to be offered to people who are the highest users.

4. Control Your Mind: Do NOT Convince Yourself That You Can Do "a Little" Drugs or Alcohol

This is a big cause of relapse, people thinking that they can do "a little" of something because they have a month or two of clean time and they think that they have got their addiction under control.

If you are an addict, you are an addict for the rest of your life and you can NEVER DO DRUGS OR ALCOHOL AGAIN, not even a little bit. This makes your situation easy to understand; zero is simple.

A little consumption will certainly lead to more consumption. It may take a few hours or a few days, but you will be back to where you were before and you will likely be in a worse place. Worse because you may try to use the same amount that you were using before you got clean, and it may be an overdose for you now that you have been clean for a month or two.

You will have invested time and energy into stopping using and detoxifying, and finding a sober home and a job, and these privileges are likely to disappear as quickly as your high. If you are an addict, be honest with yourself that YOU ARE AN ADDICT, meaning you are not able to control your consumption of drugs or alcohol. Accept this as your reality. It is the "hand that you were dealt" and "complete abstinence" is a simple concept for you to understand.

The use of one drug can quickly lead to the use of another drug. Don't fool yourself that you can smoke weed but not smoke meth or you can take a valium but not an opiate pill. One will lead to the other, and soon you will be back into your drug of choice and your pattern of addiction.

There is great relief in truly accepting absolute abstinence because you don't have to worry about hangovers, blackouts, overdoses, regulating your consumption, etc. Even if you have years of clean time, understand that if you start using again, you will be using like an addict again.

5. Control Your Mind: Do NOT Stress

Stress will increase the chances of a relapse. An addict, especially early in recovery, should not do activities, physical or mental, that cause large amounts of stress. Family, sexual relationships, money, and travel are major sources of stress for most people; try to avoid them.

To keep stress low, an addict should keep their life simple; live in a sober home, go to work and recovery meetings, and be of service to your community, while getting clean time under your belt.

Most people get stressed by the scenarios that they create in their mind, rather than the reality they are experiencing at that moment. Try to live in your immediate environment, rather than the various frightening scenarios that you can imagine. This will help you to keep your stress levels down. No NOT let your mind run wild with various scary scenarios that are unlikely to ever become true but will cause you to stress out. Control your mind; it is the key to long-term sobriety.

It is likely that at this moment you are safe, fed, watered, and reasonably comfortable. Don't panic, and don't stress out. Stress can cause a relapse, which could kill you. Take stress seriously and do all that you can to avoid it.

Chapter 5: Control Your Mind to Achieve Long-Term Sobriety

All these long-term solutions involve controlling your mind or training your brain and putting your thoughts on a leash. This is the key to long-term sobriety. Only you can do this. Other people cannot do it for you. Controlling your mind will give you freedom from your addiction and the opportunity to have a meaningful life.

In my opinion, this is what works over the long-term in recovery from addiction:

1. Control Your Mind: The Answer is LOVE!
2. Control Your Mind: Honesty Is Essential
3. Control Your Mind: Learn to Say "No"
4. Control Your Mind: Improve Your Emotional Intelligence
5. Control Your Mind: Talk about your Feeling and Actions
6. Control Your Mind: Voices and Identities
7. Control Your Mind: Be Your Own Person
8. Control Your Mind: Move toward Something New

1. Control Your Mind: The Answer Is LOVE!

The answer to all your questions is "LOVE." If you can have one attitude that will assist you more than any other, it is LOVE ALL PEOPLE and all their actions, including the "stupid stuff" they do. Love the difficulties you encounter. Love the people who have hurt you. This is difficult and it is beyond my personal ability to do this all the time, although I try to have this attitude and I find I keep re-enforcing this message to myself so that over time I am more able to feel love towards all other people.

In your journey of recovery, you will have many questions, for example, "How do I talk to my family about my recovery?" or "How do I treat my ex-lover?" The answer to these questions and all your other questions is with LOVE.

When you are focused on feeling love for everyone and everything, your brain is full of positive emotion. You are the person who feels this positive emotion more than anyone else, and it is you who benefits the most from these feelings of love.

I also recommend that you try to love yourself, not in an arrogant way. A humble, confident love for yourself is health.

Most people who are in recovery from addiction have done some nasty, stupid stuff in their addiction. Most addicts will have lied and cheated, stolen from relatives and stores, promised the world and delivered dirt. It may be hard to love yourself, so start by forgiving yourself, while not blaming others for your bad actions.

Think about the positive qualities you see in yourself. Write down your positive attributes and start building your love of yourself by loving your most positive attributes. In my opinion, you will get further faster by playing to your strengths rather than improving your weaknesses. I do not mean that you should be conceited in your love of yourself or sweep your negative actions under the carpet. I mean build a positive self-image and include yourself in your attitude of love toward all people.

Love other people for their positive qualities and ignore their negatives qualities. Other people will feel your positive vibes and return the same vibes back to you.

2. Control Your Mind: Honesty Is Essential

Being honest with yourself and others is a big part of the solution to addiction. In my own path of recovery, I have noticed myself becoming more honest with myself and with others. There seems to be layers to honesty, similar to the layers of an onion or the skill levels of a martial artist. Being honest about the amount of drugs or alcohol you are using, or were using, is a good starting point. Take an honest look at your lifestyle and how helpful you are to others in your lifestyle.

Look at your finances and your ability to make money to support yourself. Whether you like it or not, making money is a major factor in life, and everyone needs to be honest with themselves about their ability to make money.

Generally, I recommend you inform your employer you are in recovery from addiction. An employee/employer relationship is an important relationship. It should be an honest relationship and important information should not be omitted. There are exceptions to this general statement, for example, if you will lose your job by informing your employer.

I also recommend that an addict inform their employer that they have a problem with addiction if they are not yet in recovery. It is possible that the employer will have a program to help an employee with recovery from addiction and they may appreciate your honesty. If you are an airline pilot or a professional driver and you are addicted to alcohol, informing your employer is the responsible action to take. Innocent people can get killed by your chemical dependency and you MUST get help.

Honesty is not just limited to the amount of drugs you were using, money, and employment relationships. Honesty must become your backbone. It must be a central pillar on which you build yourself. Be honest with yourself first. Don't lie to yourself or betray your values! Then it will be easy to be honest with other people.

3. Control Your Mind: Learn to Say "NO"

In order to overcome addiction, you have to say "No" to drugs and alcohol. Use this as an opportunity to practice saying "No" to people and concepts. Many people are not good at saying "No" mostly because they want to be liked and they know that the other person wants to hear a "Yes" answer.

From childhood, kids cry and perform when they do not get what they want, but at some point, the child needs to grow up. There has to be a realization that you cannot have everything you want. The concept of "No" has to be learned.

It is good practice for an addict to say "No" to the requests of others if those requests are too great or too inconvenient for some reason. Polite and simple words can be used; "No, I am not available now" is far better than saying "Yes" and then not following through.

The economics of addiction are the opposite of the economics of recovery. When a drug dealer sells drugs to an addict, they are making money from the addict saying "Yes" to drugs. When an addict goes into recovery, very few people are making money from the addict's decision to say "No" to drugs.

The next time someone sings out your name with a sweet tone of voice, "Oh Johnny…," be prepared to hear them ask you for something. While they are making their request, prepare yourself to give them a polite, "No, not today, thank you." I guarantee that no one will ever sing out your name and then offer to do something for your benefit; it will always be that they are going to ask you for something. Just say, "No, not today, thank you." Saying "No" generally leaves more power in the hands of the person saying "No." Saying "Yes" generally means that you have a desire to be liked and you are seeking the approval of others.

I am not recommending that you become a grumpy person or that you never help other people; helping others is good for you, but you choose the time and place. You take control into your hands.

I also recommend that you stop trying to be liked by everyone. You put yourself at a disadvantage if you want other people to "like you." Wanting to be liked by everyone is an impossible goal; it is never going to happen and it puts you at a disadvantage where you are constantly trying to please other people or to seek their approval.

I am not recommending that you be nasty or a jerk. I recommend that you decide who you are and what your

58

goals are and that you say, "No, not today, thank you," to anything that pulls you away from your goals without feeling guilty that someone who you said "no" to is going to dislike you for saying "no" to them. The responsibility is on you to outgrow the need to be "liked" by everyone and gain the ability to say "no", especially to drugs and alcohol.

4. Control Your Mind: Improve Your Emotional Quotient (EQ)

Unlike intellectual quotient (IQ), emotional quotient (EQ) can be learned and improved. A high emotional quotient is displayed when a person does not react strongly to situations, does not "freak out" or "fly off the handle" or "blow their top" by overreacting.

Having a high emotional quotient is having a mental balance so that you can be flexible as well as resilient. Think of a person who you know who seems to handle life well, a person who stays calm, even when the road of life is bumpy. This person has a high emotional quotient. People who are "freaking out" all the time have a low emotional intelligence.

In your recovery from addiction, it is better to develop your emotional intelligence as high as possible. Read books on this subject and subscribe to YouTube channels that focus on improving your emotional intelligence. You will benefit from these efforts.

5. Control Your Mind: Talk about Your Feelings, Thoughts, and Actions

I have noticed that talking about something with other people takes power away from the subject that you are talking about. Shining a light on a subject and exposing the subject for many people to see takes power away from that subject and puts power into the minds of the people talking about the subject. My personal experience is that talking about a problem leaves me feeling lighter and less entangled with the problem.

Closing off a subject, putting it away in a dark "cupboard," and never talking about it with anyone gives that subject MORE power and makes that subject into a big deal within our minds.

Identify two or three people other than your sponsors who you respect and with whom you wish to have an honest and open relationship. Approach these people politely and ask them if it would be okay if you had a conversation with them about "your efforts to overcome your problem with addiction."

I do NOT recommend "airing your dirty laundry in public," you should NOT use Facebook to tell the world your troubles. I do NOT recommend talking to "friends in general" about your problems, unless the friend has special knowledge, because most friends will NOT know what to say and they may gossip to other friends about your problems, which may hurt your feelings.

I recommend attending recovery meetings and participating in the meetings by discussing your issues with peers who have probably faced similar issues. I also recommend professional counselors and social workers who are trained to listen and have experience guiding many other people who have faced similar problems.

6. Control Your Mind: Voices and Identities

In these paragraphs, I am NOT talking about paranoid schizophrenia or auditory hallucinations. This is an extremely serious mental health condition. If you experience this, you should call 911 and get yourself to a medical professional immediately. Here I am talking about the different voices in your head or different stories in your head.

Most people have several different voices or stories or tapes or loops that play out in their heads under specific circumstances. For example, a person may have a "voice" of anger, righteousness, vulnerability, pride, hunger, desire to be loved, beauty or the beast. The collection of your "voices" is your ego.

Take control of your relationship with these voices that can play over and over in your head when specific situations arise. By taking control of your relationship with these voices, you take control of yourself!

Turn down the volume of some of these voices, especially the voice that tells you it is "okay" to use drugs or practice your addiction behavior. Turn up the volume of voices that are healthy for you, such as your voice of love and helpfulness.

Examine which people or person comes into your mind's eye when a particular voice is playing. Which person is it who is talking? Can you visualize them? What do you like or dislike about this person? A voice or story can become so strong that it becomes one of your identities. Take control of this relationship within your mind and make this relationship work to your advantage.

You can move your center of consciousness by lowering the volume on voices that are unhealthy for you and increasing the volume of voices that are healthy for you. This is a way to take control of your life and who you are. It is a way to control how you show up in life and the content of your character. By taking control of your relationship with the voices, stories, personas or identities in your head, you can move your center of consciousness into a zone that will leave you more content. By taking control of yourself, you take control of how other people perceive you. If your center of consciousness is focused on loving others and helping others, you are likely to feel more contentment and more fulfilled with life.

Most people have multiple identities, not just one. A person may be a lover, scholar, athlete, brother or sister, son or daughter, mother or father, beast or bitch. Addicts need to control the beast or bitch within us or it will kill us by our addiction. Many people are not peaceful by nature. Human history shows many examples of extremist, violent, and self-centered behavior. Some of us also create an alcoholic or drug-addict identity. This last identity needs to disappear completely and your other identities need to be shifted around in order to facilitate the space left by the disappearance of the alcoholic or drug-addict identity.

We have all heard of the "Jekyll and Hyde" personas that are often present in a bad-tempered alcoholic. What personas do you have? Which personas do you love the most? Be more of that person.

My personal experience is that recovery has given me a greater clarity of mind, it seems that the voices in my head are on the same page or consolidated into one voice. This contributes to my feeling of contentment.

I recommend that you create the "BEST-VERSION-OF-ME" persona and live that identity as much as you can. Who you want to become is more important than who you have been! Repetition is important to make the "best-version-of-me" persona into your default persona and you practice it every day for years.

Have fun playing with this concept and be creative. The world does not need another cookie-cut persona. The world needs you with all your unique individuality, especially if you are at your best.

7. Control Your Mind: Be Your Own Person

Each person in recovery should take care of themselves first and develop their own path, in recovery and in life. When you set your own goals, values, and standards and you honestly pursue them, you will be leading by example and that will help other people.

Determining for yourself what you really want, what goals you really value, be as specific as possible. Write this information down. It is never to late to do this and now is a good time to start. It is going to take effort to achieve these goals, and if you really, really want them, you will be willing to take on the responsibility to achieve them and put in the required effort. Once you have set these goals, stop comparing yourself to other people. Only compare yourself to the person you were yesterday or a month ago.

Being your own person and following your own path is more likely to give you success in recovery and more likely to give you a meaningful life. You will still have to work hard and endure suffering because life is not easy, nor fair, but if you choose what you want to do, what your values are, and who you want to be, the suffering and hardships that you endure can be a pleasurable pain. The purpose of your life is the meaning that you give to your life, and even your death is more acceptable when you have done what you have wanted to do.

How you live your life will determine how you die. If you live your life courageously, you will die courageously. I do not mean on a battle field, I mean lying in your death bed, you will have courage as you contemplate your own death. If there is an after life, how you lived and how you died will be carried with you into your after life. Be your own person, take control of your life, don't allow addiction to define you.

What other people say or do has very little bearing on your life, except the meaning that YOU give to what other people say or do. I recommend that you pay NO attention to what other people say or do. It does not matter. What matters is WHAT YOU DO! Your actions are what are important. What you think about is important, but only to the degree that it drives your ACTIONS.

I recommend that you do things that you feel give your life purpose and meaning. Do not pursue happiness or money; pursue purpose and meaning instead. You are likely to feel more content and at peace with yourself if you are doing things that have meaning to you.

You decide what goals you consider worthy of your time. This is why you must decide your own path and be your own person. In the pursuit of the goals that you consider worthy of your time, you will find your positive emotions, your happiness.

Lead by example and do NOT seek the approval of others. I am not suggesting that you be rude to other people. Everyone deserves to be treated politely, but do not crave the approval of other people. You become more powerful when you don't need to be liked by other people.

It is important that you take responsibility for being your own person and that you lead by example. When you do this, other people will be attracted to the vibes that you are putting out and miraculously people and situations will manifest into your life without you having to forcefully find these people or situations. Good things will come your way because you have set the stage for these good things to enter your life.

It is not always possible to have a paid job that gives your life purpose and meaning. The meaningfulness of paid work can be organized into a hierarchy of job, career, passion or calling. We are lucky if we get paid to pursue our passion or calling. Sometimes it is our activities outside of work that give our life purpose. If you do these things for long enough, you may get so good at them that you get paid to do what gives your life meaning. There can be great pleasure and pride in being very good at your job or career work. Even through the work may not be your passion or calling, performing your work with a high degree of professionalism can create a meaningful life.

8. Control Your Mind: Move toward Something New

During the first six months of being clean and sober, there is an opportunity to identify new interests that you will move toward. Getting loaded is a ritual that the addict is very familiar with, and when that is removed, there is time and space that appears to be empty.

I recommend that you do not over-analyze the past. It is better to focus on your strengths and what you are going to do in the future. It is important to be adaptive. The world of today is changing rapidly and you can expect to have several "careers" and do several geographic moves. It is necessary to re-invent yourself and keep moving towards a "new and improved" version of yourself.

Perhaps you have always wanted to do stand-up comedy or play a musical instrument or learn to use a sewing machine or learn to surf. It does not matter what "blows your hair back," but it is helpful to identify some new interests or hobbies, and start moving toward them. These new interests must be important to your self-identity. They will help you to replace the part of you that identified with drug use.

I have found that surfing takes all my land-based troubles away from me. I focus on the waves and the water, and when I come back to land, I feel refreshed. Not everyone wants to go surfing, but you may have an activity that you do or want to do that has a similar effect on you.

In my opinion, fear should be INCLUDED in the interests that you move toward. It is possible that people who are willing to try drugs are more adventurous than most people and a hobby or interest that involves some fear is a healthy alternative to your old habits. I am NOT recommending that you take up activities that "scare the hell" out of you; just a little bit of fear is what I recommend, enough so that you have to control your mind in order to control your fear so that you can do the activity. In my opinion, people benefit from confronting their fears. If you identify what makes you fearful and move toward it, it makes you more powerful. Overcoming your fear can help to create a healthy mindset.

As you move toward something new, I recommend that you DRESS differently than you did in the past! I live on the same property as my clients and I see some of them dress as if they were still using drugs or alcohol. There are standard methods of dressing for addicts—both men and woman—that are almost a uniform. For example, a man wearing long white socks up to the knees, baggy pants worn below their bum, with their underwear showing, and a dirty off-white "wife-beater" vest or a black hoodie and baseball cap. This clothing screams "drug addict" and this uniform should to be replaced with a fresh, healthy look. Physically changing your clothing helps to create a better mindset.

Your clothes should be washed regularly, as well as your body. You should have a haircut and pamper your body with nice-smelling deodorants or other beauty products. Thrift stores sell clothes at inexpensive prices. There is no need to spend big money on changing your outward appearance, but making these outward changes will support the internal changes that you are making.

Reinforce your mental changes with actions, such as going to recovery meetings, dressing well, grooming yourself, talking like a productive member of society and not like a gangster selling drugs; walk upright, stand tall, keep your chin up, and put a big wide smile on your face regularly.

Moving toward something new will help you to move away from your old habits. Embrace the journey. Be playful with these changes. You can have fun and experiment. Be your heroic-self. What "super-powers" would you have? Move in that direction.

Case Study: Sterling, Skateboarding on Heroin

Sterling is 34 years old. He is married with two children and works as an electrician. He has been addicted to heroin primarily and has four years clean.

Sterling, please tell us how your addiction got started?

A lot of people believe they're born addicts, but I don't believe I was. I had parents who were addicts, and I feel that my addiction came in later years due to the decisions I made through my early years as a teenager. I started smoking weed with all my friends, skateboarding, and partying with all the kids from school. I will say that I feel like I always abused and used drugs to the extreme. The addiction that I see, whether I had the obsession to use, over all other aspects of my life, didn't come about until I was about 21 years old, when I started using heroin.

I'm curious if the people you were using with early-on if you distinguished a difference in how you used versus how they used?

There were different groups of people who would use on a school night. They used all through the night and kept going. I was definitely one of those people. There are other people who would be in between that. I didn't do that great in school. I didn't have opportunities to go to college right out of high school. I felt that I was an athlete, and I wanted to be a professional skateboarder; aspects of that life became drinking, partying, and skateboarding. Then when I got hooked on opiates, I tore my ACL. I had no money for surgery and no insurance. I sat around, trying to recover, and I did a lot of drugs. I came upon heroin, and I don't remember ever stopping, until I finally got clean four years ago.

Was it the physical pain relief that led you to heroin initially or were there other factors at play?

At first, the brain convinces you you're going to keep doing it because it's a pain reliever. I was hooked on opiates the first time I ever did them. I woke up the next morning and wanted to do it again and again. I remember the first time getting dope sick I didn't even know it was a thing. I called my friend like "What's wrong with me?" He told me, "You're dope sick. You did heroin for 14 days in a row." I was like "I'm not going to do that." But that never happened. That was the first time I told myself I was going to quit. But I didn't do what I said I was going to do. I've always held that part of it like it's a secret life.

I've been married to my wife for the last 13 years. I have a 12-year-old daughter and an eight-year-old son. I did everything to throw that thing away in order to get more dope. I had the greatest intention to get clean, to stop doing what I was doing. I had to do everything I promised my wife about getting a job and quitting, but I wasn't able to do it. My wife and I have known each other since second grade. We've been best friends since age 15 and we got married and had kids at 22. True love and soul mates, and it got so bad that she was done with me. Fortunately, that's what it takes sometimes to get people clean. Fortunately for me, I was able to get her back, but a lot of people go too far. I went too far, but I was able, through my recovery, to gain back some trust.

It doesn't sound like she dealt with addiction issues for herself. Do you think there were elements of enabling, that maybe she didn't recognize how severe your problem had become right away? How long did it go on? How long was it a serious problem for you and maybe she didn't recognize how serious it was?

I was very much in denial about my problem, so I sounded very convincing to her that I didn't have a problem. I would say that my wife liked to party. She did stuff. When life showed up, she got married and had kids; she was able to not do anything anymore but go to work and go to school. But I wasn't able to do that. She was convinced for probably four or five years that I was going to hold these promises of going back to school or getting a job and paying a bill. It was about five years of not willing to admit that she knew until she was finally convinced by her parents and friends that I was a piece of crap and that I needed to go. By all means, I did not do anything that a father and a husband should do to his family. Finally, she kicked me out. She still loved me and it was the hardest thing for her to do. She let me live in the back shed, but I couldn't see the kids. She made me crash there because she was worried about me. She didn't want me out on the streets, since I was addicted, and she didn't want me to die.

How are you taking? Were you shooting at this point or were you smoking it?

For the longest time, I was mainly a smoker. I'd go through spurts of shooting. Then I'd get over it to smoke and then I started mixing speed, meth, and heroin together. At the end, I was definitely shooting a lot more. I always was mixing it up. I wasn't just a shooter or a smoker at the end. Being out of my family's house, I was in denial. I'd finally come to terms and knew I was an addict. But I couldn't stop. Hundreds of times I had plenty of dope to go off in the morning. I'm like "I'm over it. I'm going to use everything I have tonight. Tomorrow, I'm going to wake up clean. I'm not going to do it again."

I would be at the dope man's house before I even remembered telling myself that the night before. Completely going against everything that I knew I wanted, I had the utmost intention to do these things, but there was some obsession, something in my mind that I couldn't stop. I couldn't hold the promises to the ones I love the most. Back to where I would take my kids, they copped out. It's a weird thing to say, but I was a way better parent loaded than when I was dope sick. When I was dope sick, I didn't give a crap. For me, I wasn't getting high; I was just getting not sick. It was that bad.

Did your kids have any idea? How did you hide it from them?

I walked myself into the bathroom and into the bedroom. They were so young they would see the tinfoil, not knowing what it was. I was able to hide it and lie to them. I'm sure when my son gets older if he ever sees something like that he'd be like, as a kid, "I didn't know my dad was smoking joints. When I started smoking joints, I realized that's what he was doing." My son was too young. My daughter was eight when I got clean. Back to what got me clean, how bad did it get? I'd come to terms that I was an addict. I wanted to get clean, but my family and friends had helped me already. I was like "I don't need help, but I'll do it because you say I need it." When I wanted it and needed it, they weren't there for me. I wasn't eligible for any type of program through insurance. We didn't have medical. My wife had an income and I didn't. I became suicidal, but I didn't want to die. I wanted to kill the person I'd become, a lying, cheating, and thieving person. I just want that person to be gone.

I thought the only way was to take my life. It was such an intense thought that I tried to intentionally overdose. Fortunately, I can't afford it because my addiction levels and my body were so saturated with the drug. I had written a letter to my wife and it scared her. She woke me up in the back shed and said, "I'm going to call the cops." She'd called the Suicide Hotline. I didn't know it was a thing and she had gotten advice. She was like "He needs a program. If he goes to the emergency room and signs a 5150, he's instantly eligible for mental health funding." She brought that by me

73

and said, "If you don't go to the hospital, I'm going to call the Sheriff's and they will take you." I have this letter. It was to help me. I look at it this way, while in recovery, we talked about a higher power, and before that, I hadn't been willing to look into that, or even if one was working in my life, be able to recognize it.

I was in the program within three days. Instantly, I was getting that low, hitting that bottom, and getting suicidal, and all the things that happened were definitely a higher power working my life, trying to save it. I didn't get clean at that time. I had 30 days, but I didn't work the program. It was the first time where the recovery was planned when I knew and went to the rooms of Narcotics Anonymous. I saw people getting clean. I saw people's lives changing. It gave my wife hope, and then I pissed it all away again.

About eight months later, she made me leave the house again after I came back. She thought I had a whole 90 days. I lied. Being an addict, I was a very good manipulator. She wanted the father of her children and her best friend since age 15 and husband for nine years to get clean; she had that hope. She asked me to leave again eight months later when I couldn't hide anything any longer. I couldn't lie about anything anymore.

How strong and messed up my addiction was, I should have been even sadder and depressed. She was gone. She said she was divorcing me. Something told me like "I don't have to lie about it anymore. I can use. I don't have to hide it." A very short time later, I told myself I had enough of heroin, and if I would have enough not to get dope sick, I'd be able to go to work and hold that job. I wouldn't have to disappear and wait for the dope man for four hours and she'd be like "Where were you?" Not coming home with dope money or the milk.

I ended up coming upon a large portion of money, totally randomly, in my dad's garage. He was asleep one night and I found a check from my grandma, who had passed away, for $3,000. I wasn't living at home. That was over. I knew I was going to be a dealer now. I was selling heroin. I was in my dad's garage again.

But I was more miserable than before. I had all the dope and I thought I was going to be okay. I knew I'd never had that before. I didn't have to worry about getting sick and doing things. I was so miserable and over my life, my mom called me. But prior to this, my mom would not have anything to do with me. She would see the kids on Christmas. She was mad at my wife for not kicking me out sooner. She had done some research on heroin and how it hijacks your brain. She wanted to help me. I was like "I'm over this. I need help. I don't want to do this." She called, "higher power, this is your chance." She's like "I know you're homeless. I know she's divorcing you. Come up to Sausalito, and I will get you into a program. I will pay for it and we will help you."

My addict brain kicked back in. I got two ounces of dope. I was straight up with my mom. I was selling dope and I said to her, "Can I sell it all first and then come up there?" She said, "Flush it and I will take care of you." I flushed a lot of it. I told her that I flushed it all. I hid a bunch in my ass. My brother came with another addict in the program and I didn't know if he was clean. He was coming to try and come up on my stuff. He had met me at a Xanax bar and I had been up for a while. At that point, mixing speed and heroin, I blacked out, and they went through all my stuff, found the rest of it, and got rid of it for me. When I woke up at her house in Sausalito, it was February 1 and I've been clean since that day. It's a weird thing and I've talked about this with my sponsor in Narcotics Anonymous many times. I know I wanted my mommy. I don't use that word, mommy—"I want my mom"—I hadn't had that for 10 years.

I was very jealous of my wife and her mom's relationship. I would make fun of her for it. But In reality I wanted that same thing. I had something and I call it hope. I hadn't had that for a long time. I had previously, eight months earlier. I had been introduced to meetings and a program. I knew where to go. In the beginning, I went to the rooms of Alcoholics Anonymous. I jumped right in. I got a sponsor. I did everything they said. I would recommend this to people who have struggled trying to get clean. What I did at first was VIVITROL, a 30-day opiate-blocker. I did 60 days of it, along with some therapy and drug counseling. It gave me confidence. VIVITROL is a 30-day time-released injection in the muscle on your butt. It blocks your opioid receptors so that you can get high if you want to. I've heard of people trying it, and I've also heard people say it works really well. But I had to find out for myself. They wanted me to take it for a year.

The hope that I've gotten, the clear-headedness, but I didn't want people giving credit to something else. They are like "It's a good thing you did VIVITROL." I would say, "It's a good thing I did in the beginning, but I was doing what I was told by my sponsor and other people in recovery who were staying clean and getting lives worth living." I stopped taking it against my parents' advice. I kept getting lots of commitments in Alcoholics Anonymous.

I want to jump back to my wife. She was very relieved I was in a safe place, and she didn't have to worry about me. In my mind, i was like "I'm going to fix this. I'm going to save it." But I was in denial about how far gone I was. She wanted me to come sign divorce papers. I didn't do it for a while. It was hard for me. I want people to know they can stay clean through absolutely everything.

It's a weird higher-power thing. I like music and it was weird because I didn't listen to any new music. I didn't even know what a smartphone was. I had this thing called Pandora. You put in one artist you like. I played this song, "You Only Love Her If You Let Her Go." I don't remember who did it. I'm looking for meaning in life at this point in my life. If I love her, I've got to let it go. Then immediately after it comes on, a Jack MJJ song that we danced to at our wedding, "Better Together," comes on, and that was my sign that I had to try and make things work. I had to not sign those papers and give up because I had never felt this before. I never felt the hope that I can stay clean and change my life. It's weird when I say I look for things. If those songs would have come on in reverse order, I may have gone the other way, our song, and then that song.

I rushed down to Santa Cruz. It's about an hour and 10 minutes away from where I was at. I had to get some clothes and some other things. She was wearing makeup. She's an all-natural girl who doesn't usually wear a lot of makeup. I looked at her. I was like "You're beautiful—what do you need makeup for?" She started crying. I knew it right away. I was like "Are you seeing somebody?" We had talked about it and we were going to wait for the divorce to be finalized before we saw other people.

Instantly, my addict mind jumped in and I said, "I can't believe you." Then in that recovery voice that I was slowly starting to learn, I said, "I was cheating on you for so long with heroin and drugs and on your heart and not being able to be there for you emotionally." She was emotionally lonely for so long, so I told her, "It's okay. I love you and I'm not signing these papers. This is totally way out of my character." She said that was the first time she had seen the changed me.

"I'm not flipping out," I said. I got in my car and drove immediately out of Santa Cruz, where I was used to using. I called my sponsor. I lost it then. I was crying and then a powerful song came on the radio. I can get through this, I thought, and then I stopped crying. Then a sad song came on; it was on the country station. Then I was bawling like a little girl.

In the beginning, I said, "You can make it through anything." To me, that was the most painful thing I ever felt. Calling my sponsor and him telling me, "This will pass. If you go use drugs or alcohol, you will only make it worse." I believed him. I kept going to meetings. I worked the steps through it. She had seen that change in me too. I still didn't want to give up. I got a job. I started giving her money. I had never done that. In the 10 years of being addicted, and living with her, I'd give her only a few bucks here or there. The paychecks always disappeared and not make it home with me. But now I'm sending my wife money. I'm giving her money and paying bills.

What work were you doing?

Any construction work I could do. Most jobs before using were stuff I'd get paid for at the end of the day. Somehow, during those 10 years, I had gone to an electrical trade school and I was able to graduate, through cheating, even though I was out through half of the class. I'm a smart person, just fully hindered by my addiction. I took the world up on what I got and I went to a company in San Jose called Sunrun Solar Company and I applied. They hired me as a ground-level installer. I worked my butt off for four months and then another six months after that.

It's by showing up, the things I learned, and through the program, through having commitments. I showed up every time 15 minutes earlier, and you don't want to be the first one to leave. I had a job and I had insurance through my job that I could put my kids and her on. Not just my kids, because she was divorcing me still. I ended up telling her I can't keep dragging her along. I have to let her go. I told her, "I will sign those divorce papers for you only after you let me take you out on one last date, and if you don't feel something or want to change after that, I'll sign the papers for you." In my mind, I didn't think I was going to sign these papers. I was so convinced that it was going to work, that I was going to do something. I planned the most amazing date. I got Stub Hub on my phone. You've got to think I'd never had a credit card or a debit card or a smartphone. I was never able to do these things. Life was so new. It was like being a little kid and exploring nature

I got these tickets to this awesome show. We used to go to a bunch of raves, electronic music shows back in the day before we were married and before my heroin addiction. I found this new artist and they were playing at the Berkeley Greek Theater. I planned this awesome dinner and picnic. It was like the most amazing thing ever. When we got back, I dropped her off. I turned my eyes in the room and said, "What do you want to do?" Every inch of her body was telling her not to. I'd let her down so many times. I had given that promise I am going to do what it takes. I've changed and I wasn't using. I let her down so many times in the past. Something in her seemed to change that I had felt in myself. She said, "We can hold off on signing the papers. I definitely see that change, but you need to move back to Santa Cruz and stay clean for a period of time before I know and I see it's real."

In the program, they tell you if you're fully geographic, you are likely to find the same thing. But she didn't know that little saying. And she thought because I was in a protected area somewhere else, but there is dope everywhere right next to San Francisco. So I could have gotten it if I wanted it. I was like "Whatever you want." That's when I called a friend in Narcotics Anonymous and told him I needed to get into a sober living environment in Santa Cruz. That's how I got introduced to Gault House Sober Living Environment, which took me in immediately. When you first move into a sober living environment, there is a strict curfew and you need to get a job. I already had all that and I had people in the program. I definitely can give credit to this house. (Gault House is a recovery residence for men and women who choose to live together free from illicit drugs and alcohol and addictive behavior.)

What was it like getting back into your wife's life, and likewise? What about getting back into your kids' lives?

It was a hard thing at first because my wife and I had to tell them about we're getting divorced. We held it off so long I ignored that we're getting divorced and I ignored about the kids. I still felt that there was a chance. I didn't want to admit it to them that it was over for sure. I can't even explain what it was like to be a father. It came so quick and natural. I had patience for them. They took me back like I was never gone. There was something different. I can't explain it, but they responded to me much differently. Kids are very intuitive. They definitely realize Mom and Dad are fighting. You're a king or a God to them. You are Dad or you are Mom and you trust them no matter what. I broke that trust with them without them knowing. Getting back in their lives has been an amazing thing. I'm currently at a spot where I had never imagined being.

I lived at Gault House for a while and then my wife let me move back in. I kept paying bills and I kept showing up and I had to explain to them my recovery. Early recovery is especially intense. In recovery, the first thing you put in your recovery is the first thing you'll lose. I don't want to risk this gift that I'd been given recently that I thought I would never have. Three or four months later, I planned an amazing tenth wedding anniversary for my wife and I in Hawaii.

We had gone to Hawaii on our honeymoon. I paid for it. But I didn't take her on one trip 10 years after that. I secretly talked to her mom, which is also the biggest deal that I've been able to get their trust back. I asked her mom, since she worked for her mom, "Can she have these 10 days off? I'm taking her to Hawaii for our tenth wedding anniversary." We went. I told her two weeks before. She's a jeweler. She personally designed a new wedding ring for me because I had been an addict, doping, trying to get dope at all costs. I definitely got rid of my wedding ring. I pawned it. I'm going to buy it back, I thought. But I never got the $40 to buy it back from the pawnshop and I lost it.

She had made a new one for me and gave it to me when we hit the beach in Hawaii. When we got back from Hawaii, we burnt the divorce papers together in the barbecue pit. It's like the happily ever after story. I realized that a lot of people don't get that back, that it's too late. Even if you lose that someone, your life can be brought back to you by staying and doing the next great thing.

Currently, I can say that the best thing for me in recovery is to be reliable and honest and people can trust me. I don't want to be a liar and I didn't have to lie. My wife told me one day, "I never lied to you. You're my husband; I never lied to you. But you lied to me every day." That hurt. But I'm never going to lie to her again.

If you ever go to your 10-year reunion as an addict, you need to know most addicts won't probably make it. You see these people are doing amazing things with their lives, becoming men. I'm like "I had missed out on that. I wasn't a man." They say you don't mature when you're using. It was definitely my story. It was so exciting to start to grow up and be a man at 31 years old. But I still do my meetings. I still have a sponsor.

My life is so full and busy. Sometimes I joke when I do chairs in AA meetings saying, "Sometimes I wish I could go back to rehab." It's such a safe place. They'll feed you three square meals a day. You don't have to worry about any of the outside life. They'll wipe your ass for you. I always tell the people, "Take advantage of this," and I'm like "I'm stoked to be here. I'm in a safe place. I'm into recovery." If you stay clean, life shows up and gets busy. I'm a commercial foreman for an electrical company. I'm about ready to pass my journeyman's test for electrical. I'm getting ready to buy a house with my wife in Santa Cruz through the help of her parents. To be able to have that trust and that type of life that they see that it's worth investing in and it's a big deal.

The biggest thing for me and my new passion in life is coaching little kids. My son is eight years old. He is a very advanced baseball player. I get to manage his baseball teams. I'm on the board for the Little League. It's a big part of my life. They say get commitments and give back. I'm not just giving back to my Narcotics Anonymous program, I'm also giving back to the community, from which I stole and for which I was not a productive member of for so long. I see a really crazy story. I was coaching this little kid. I reached out and grabbed his arms. I looked over at this guy's dad in there and he was a cop who had arrested me before. This kid was not listening to me and he goes, "Listen to Coach." He yelled it across the field. I thought he recognized me. I looked so different that I don't think he recognized me.

People trust me with their kids. Coaching is an amazing feeling. Little kids call you Coach. When I was in my addiction, I walked down the street, hitting the side of the road with a baseball bat. I don't run a perfect program through Narcotics Anonymous, but the only thing I do is I absolutely do not put stuff in my body. And it changed the way I feel. I've got a lot of friends who I can call. I've never had a real desire to use since I lost it. I thought I would, but I'd keep doing the next right thing.

I can say over the last four years I've literally been on a perpetual pink cloud. My first sponsor was a short Jewish gangster guy, who said, "You can live on a pink cloud as long as you build yourself a pink elevator." He taught me how to do that and I do that. I have lots of goals written down, little ones and big ones, like graduate from college. That's a tedious task and it takes years. You get down to yourself, trying to do that, and accomplish your goal.

He taught me, "Go pay that ticket at the DMV." Do all these little things that as addicts we would not do. Do the little things and have it be like a planning process. When you do it, you feel good about yourself. I've literally written multiple pages of goals and I crossed them off and redone it. I didn't accomplish a goal my entire using.

I love sayings. People out there in early recovery say, "Don't count the days; make the days count." That is one of my favorite sayings that hit me in recovery. It's like day 28, 29, 30. My next saying is "I live my recovery not by sitting in the rooms of the 12-Step programs and waiting for life to happen to me; I have to actively go out and create a life that's worth living." My favorite saying is from Abraham Lincoln that goes, "Good things come to those who wait, but only the things left by those who go out and get it."

I go out and get life and show up. I help other people. I definitely do not deserve the life that I've been given. The person I am now, I deserve what I get. It's hard to look back on the things that I've done and go, "This is what he used to be and this is what he gets now. Why?" I can't explain why. It's a tough thing to think about drugs. Seeing friends out there, I was like "Why don't they even get it?" You want to go out and rescue them and bring them in. I just helped.

His mom called me and some other friends who don't use had called me and asked me to talk to him. I gave him my best pitch. I looked him in the eye when he wouldn't look me in the eye. He was so loaded and so in denial, as I said, "Let me help you." He pulled out of there. But in my eyes, he needed it. People are dying out there. But he was like "Why not me? I wanted to die."

What advice would you give to somebody in the in the same situation as your friend who's maybe considering recovery? It sounds to me you had a lot of motivation to help push you into recovery. Do you think everybody needs that in order to find it? What advice would you give to somebody who's struggling with that idea?

When I took that first step of the 12 Steps and I fully admitted I was an addict, a weight was lifted off my shoulders. I fought it for so long. I always wanted to believe I was a smart person. I felt like if I surrendered and admitted I was an addict then that meant I was dumb. Someone gave me another good saying: "Surrender isn't weakness. It is being smart enough to know when you've been defeated, so that you can live to fight another day." My friend's mom was supporting him; he was a codependent. For me, what happened was, as soon as my wife didn't love me anymore, it sent me down to that pit of despair much faster.

I feel like I don't want everyone to have to hit that rock bottom like I did. I wish I knew what it was that convinced somebody before they get there. I do hear about people who don't have to hit a very big bottom, that maybe their lives were a lot better in the beginning, so they don't have to go as far down. It's hard to tell. All I can say is go to a meeting, talk to someone. I didn't know anything about life, so I literally had to find someone who did. I wanted to change. I didn't know how to get it, so I did what I was told. They say do what your sponsor does, do what they tell you. It's a hard thing. If you're thinking about recovery, then maybe come to terms with that you are an addict and that you need help. You're not going to get any worse by trying.

What was your biggest takeaway from all your experiences until now when using led to your recovery? What was the biggest lesson you learned for yourself?

I truly believe that everything happens for a reason—the person I'm becoming and continuously growing into. I feel like everything was a lesson and that it has created the person who I am. I love who I am now. Maybe things wouldn't be the same. I have the most amazing kids. Maybe they wouldn't be the same people if I hadn't been using. Honesty is a big thing. Friends can call me and say, "Help me move." If I say, 'I'm going to be there," they know I'm going to be there. The biggest lesson I've gotten from recovery is how to be honest and be accountable, and not push everything off on everyone else and not blame the world. I literally love my life and that's a hard thing to come to terms with sometimes. When I look where I'm at and I see people in recovery, and I was there, it's hard to see that I was there. Sometimes becoming the person I've become, I realize it doesn't happen to everyone that quick.

Sometimes you've got more court problems to deal with. You've done damage to your loved ones too. It's unfortunate that the people we hurt the most are the people who we love the most. I'd say my favorite thing about recovery is growth. I am constantly growing. I'm not the same person I was a month ago. I've learned new things about myself, growing and becoming a man, because for so long, I hadn't been growing. My wife had grown so much over those 10 years. I pondered over it. It was a messed-up feeling like you're going to be one of those old dudes. "Back in my day"—that's stupid. My deepest, darkest secret now is that I was listening to Taylor Swift. My daughter left the CD in my car and it came on. And I left it on. I was rocking out to that open-mindedness. It's a crazy little thing that I had never experienced before.

That's a remarkable story, Sterling. I want to thank you for sharing it with us. I want to thank our readers for joining us. To all of you, including you, Sterling, we wish you to stay sober and be happy. Take care.

Thanks.

Chapter 6: Mental Health Needs Funding

Mental health and drug addiction are closely related. Excessive drug use induces mental health issues and many people with mental health issues are attracted to use drugs to mask their mental health issues or to find relief from them. Someone who has detoxed for a week from drug use has not fixed any underlying mental health issues that caused them to be attracted to drugs or alcohol in the first place. These mental health issues can be mild to very serious.

Anyone wanting to overcome addiction must address their mental health and any underlying issues. I do NOT recommend talking to "friends" about your mental health. I recommend using professional counselors, social workers, and psychologists. These people are trained to listen and trained to help others with mental health problems. These resources are available even if you have very little or no money. If you look for this type of professional help, you will find it.

Mental health is a broad subject. In this chapter, I look at a few areas of mental health that I have had experiences with while running a sober home:

1. What Came First, the Mental Health Problem or Drug Addiction?
2. Bi-Polar Is Difficult in a Sober Home
3. Suicide Is a Domestic Tragedy
4. Post-Traumatic Stress Disorder Is Common
5. Adult Child: Arrested Development Is Common

1. What Came First, the Mental Health Problem or Drug Addiction?

Mental health and drug addiction are closely related. One leads to the other, and vice versa. A large percentage of people with mental health problems also have drug addiction problems and many people who use drugs regularly develop mental health problems because of their regular drug use. There are many examples where a drug addict did not have mental health problems, but their frequent use of heavy drugs caused mental health issues. Heavy use of meth will induce paranoid schizophrenia. Frequent use of a cocktail of heavy drugs will scramble your ability to think.

Modern life is complicated and there are disappointments on many levels; some are small and some are big. There are reasons to feel down about life and depression is common. Most clients who come to our sober home from a drug rehab center will have been prescribed an antidepressant medication because a medical professional licensed to prescribe drugs has decided that the mental health of our client could benefit from the assistant that these drugs can provide.

Depression and anxiety are common for people in early recovery and the prescribing of antidepressants and anti-anxiety medications are also common. In my opinion, people should follow the advice of their doctors and people should also try to get off ALL drugs and not start any new drug unless it was absolutely necessary.

Whether the drug is a prescription drug or an illicit drug, people turn to chemicals for relief from mental anguish and their real problems do not get addressed. If the underlying problems are never addressed, the pattern of using chemicals for relief normally gets worse. The long-term result is a mental health patient with a drug-addiction problem. It is difficult to know which problem came first, the mental health problems or the drug addiction problem. Consider this example; a paranoid schizophrenic with a history of violence using heroin to subdue himself and then detoxing from heroin. Does this person have a mental health problem or a drug addiction problem or both?

Mental health patients are generally treated with compassion by society, while drug addicts receive very little support by comparison. In the short term, it costs society more money to care for a mental health patient than a drug addict. The mental health patient is normally housed in a secure hospital-style setting. There are plenty of trained staff and program administrators to take care of the patient, and meals are served three times a day. It costs approximately $10,000 per month to house and treat a mental health patient, and the cost is paid for by a combination of family and government programs.

Drug addicts and alcoholics, by comparison, are demonized and kicked to the curb, dismissed as "no good," and given very little support. There is no budget to accommodate all the drug addicts and alcoholics within the mental health programs. Neither family members nor government programs can afford to accommodate all the mental health applicants in professionally managed mental health facilities. The most severe mental health patients are accommodated within the mental health programs and all the rest get pushed out into society. Many people who are mental health patients find themselves living in sober homes, thinking they are drug addicts in recovery, but their problems are bigger than that. The pricing structure of a sober home is low (approximately $1,000 per month per person), but this price does not include full-time attendance by nursing staff, administrators, social workers, and mental health professionals. Consequently, many sober homes are dealing with mental health patients without the resources to do so, and the long-term cost to society is much higher.

For example, at our sober home we had a client viciously attacked another client over a small dispute. The assailant called 911 to report his actions and request an ambulance. Fortunately, the victim lived, but the assailant was charged with attempted murder by the District Attorney and he is likely to go to jail for five years or more. Then the jail will be housing a mental health patient with a drug-addiction problem. There is a strong argument that this assailant should never have been in a sober home in the first place, and had he been in a mental health facility, he would not be headed for jail in the near future. This attack was a surprise to everyone because the assailant seemed to be a laid-back stoner dude with a hippie attitude. Only two hours before the attack, he was tested for drugs and alcohol and he had neither in his system.

Whatever the underlying causes are for his actions, this is an example where a mental health patient ended up in a sober home because there is no money to fund their stay in an appropriate mental health facility. The "can" gets kicked down the road and is dealt with by a sober home that was never intended or designed to be dealing with this type of problem. If we treat drug addicts as mental health patients rather than criminals, our society with benefit and it will cost less in the long run.

I recommend that all drugs and alcohol be legalized and mandatory registration be required in order to access these substances. This way, drug addicts can register and receive the drugs they crave, as well as services to help them.

2. Bi-Polar Is Difficult in a Sober Home

A "bi-polar" condition seems like a relatively easy condition to deal with at first glance. The term bi-polar implies that a person is happy some of the time and sad some of the time. However, a bi-polar diagnosis has a spectrum of severity and the happy/sad patient is at the entry point of the spectrum. In my experience, bi-polar clients have been some of the most difficult clients for our sober home to accommodate. Many bi-polar clients prefer one of their mood states over the other, so they end up not taking their medication or over-medicating in order to stay in their preferred mood stage, either manic (high energy) or sad (depressed).

A bi-polar client who is not taking their medication and not seeing a doctor regularly so that they get the right medications, at the right levels, is a major problem for a sober home. Their mood swings leave other people in the home not knowing how to interact with the bi-polar client and consequently the bi-polar person gets ignored and becomes isolated within a group setting. This leads the bi-polar person to act out and either over-medicate or under-medicate, and the management of the sober house has to give a disproportionate amount of attention to the bi-polar client.

There are many prescription drugs that are acceptable within a sober home (see the chapter entitled "Drugs Most Commonly Used, Illicit and Medically Assisted Treatment"), but I prefer to run a sober home as a "drug-free home," as much as possible. A bi-polar patient is typically taking a large amount of medications to manage their up-side and to manage the down-side and some of these medications can be abused by other clients. This make a bi-polar client a poor fit for a sober home.

3. Suicide Is a Domestic Tragedy

There are approximately 50,000 suicides every year in the United States. For comparison, 2,977 Americans lost their life in the September 11, 2001, attacks and 58,300 Americans lost their life in the 21 years of the war in Vietnam. This suicide rate equates to approximately 132 people killing themselves each day, or approximately one person killing themselves every 10 minutes. According to statistics available on the Internet, there are 20 attempted suicides for every successful suicide. This means that every 30 seconds, someone in America tries to kill themselves. These numbers are staggeringly high and they are not likely to turn downward in the near future.

Drug addiction and alcoholism puts people in a higher-risk category for suicide. When an addict or alcoholic is deep into their addiction, they feel isolated, lonely, depressed, and unwanted, and to a large degree, they are right. Western society, both the government and the general public, treat drug addicts and alcoholics as low-status individuals. There are very few people who care about these people.

At our sober home, there have been no suicides or attempted suicides that we know of, but there have been several clients who have lost siblings to suicide. Is this coincidence or do drug addiction and mental health issues run in the family?

Suicide is mostly a mental health issue and I believe that drug addiction and alcoholism are also mostly a mental health issue. There are many examples of addicts who have committed suicide. What names come to your mind? Robin Williams, the world-famous comedian and actor, is a good example of a drug addict and alcoholic who's mental health deteriorated and he committed suicide. There are many others.

4. Post-Traumatic Stress Disorder (PTSD) Is Common

Post-Traumatic Stress Disorder (PTSD) is a term that originated in the 1980s. From my layman's perspective, this term was primarily used to describe mental health problems faced by soldiers who were exposed to severe stress in battle. The First World War was a bloodily war that was fought in muddy trenches with mortars, poisonous gas, and hand-to-hand combat. The soldiers who survived that war to return to "normal" civilian life were described as "shell-shocked." My grandfather was one of them, and the family said, "He was never the same again." These poor people were expected to suffer in silence, tough it out, and get on with it. That was the standard of care of that time and people lived miserable unproductive lives because of it. Not all combat veterans suffer PTSD but it is common. Addiction and suicide is more likely within this population demographic.

Now we realize that there are many situations where PTSD applies. There can be traumatic stress in everyday life and even sports. One of our clients worked as a paramedic and she was traumatized by taking down an 18-year-old girl who had committed suicide by hanging herself. Responding to paramedic calls of suicide by gunshot did not have the same effect on our client as suicide by hanging, which became impossible for her to deal with. This is an example of post-traumatic stress disorder (PTSD), and I know that counseling therapy helped our client.

During winter in Santa Cruz, California, the ocean waves get 20 to 30 feet high. Less than an hour's drive north of Santa Cruz is the famous big wave surf spot called Mavericks, where the waves can get to 50 feet high. Huge mountains of water break with a heavy lip that can snap a surfboard as if it were a pencil and these waves sometimes kill people. Highly skilled expert surfers are drawn to surf these waves; just like in other sports, people are drawn to perform their sport at the highest levels.

Surfing these huge waves can cause traumatic stress. The fear of dying is ever present. The water is cold and there is no protection against sharks. Catching a mountain of water and riding one of these waves is very exciting. It can be difficult for people to come down from the high of this type of situation. The same can be said for people playing other intense sports such as football, basketball, rugby, especially at the highest levels, where large crowds of people are cheering them on. In modern society, there are many extreme activities and many participants. Being a stock market trader or an emergency ward surgeon is extreme activity. Being a musician playing to a big audience of ecstatic fans is extreme.

Often the participants in these extreme activities choose to not come down from the natural high, preferring to stay high with the use of drugs. A couple of years of natural highs, combined with chemical highs, and society has another person with a drug addiction problem as well as a mental health problem. There are numerous famous surfers who are examples of this. The same is true for professional athletes (and amateur athletes, but we don't hear about them because they are not famous enough to make the "news"). Rock star musicians are almost expected to have a drug addiction problem, but the general public is more surprised when a clean-cut athlete is arrested for drug use. There are many examples, Tiger Woods comes to my mind. Can you think of any?

Our sober home has had many clients who are struggling with PTSD as part of their mental health issues at the same time as struggling to overcome an addiction. In my experience, PTSD is common.

5. Adult Child: Arrested Development Is Common

Drugs and alcohol contribute to a percentage of our population not maturing into productive members of our society. To varying degrees, there is a child's mind inside an adult's body. This is a mental health concern rather than a physiological concern. The cost to society is huge. Many deaths, fights, accidents, and single parenthood are due to the immaturity of the participants. Alcohol and drugs are leading many of these participants to believe that they are more mature and ready for the responsibilities of life than what they are.

Our society's approach to demonizing drugs has driven the drug trade underground, into the hands of criminals who have no concern for the welfare of the people that are buying the drugs. This has removed our society's ability to be an influencer in the decisions of the drug addict in general. With alcohol, society has gone the other way, making alcohol widely available and easy to get. Neither of these approaches is good.

I recommend that all drugs be legalized and mandatory registration be required in order to access these drugs. This way, drug addicts can register and receive the drugs they crave, as well as services to help them. In addition, I recommend that all alcohol purchases should be tracked on a centralized database. If we treat drug addicts and alcoholics as mental health patients rather than criminals, our society with benefit and it will cost our society less in the long run.

Case Study: Hayley: Mental Health, PTSD, Alcohol & Cocaine

In this episode of Stories of Addiction, I will be talking with Hayley about her addiction and her recovery from addiction.

Hi, Hayley, welcome to Responsible Recovery. It's nice to have you here. How did your addiction start?

If you were to ask me how my addiction started before, it would be the last two years, but when I look back on my life, it started when I was young. It didn't manifest as drugs or alcohol when I was super-young, but it manifested as different things. I grew up a privileged little kid. It was a great family. My parents had been married for 41 years. I was always that curious, rebellious little kid who would get all my work done and talk in school and interrupt people. As a little kid, it was very obvious. My mom would say, "You're just a 36-year-old version of your three-year-old self." She always said that. I always was looking for a way to break the rules or get attention in a different way. I was always outside of myself my whole life when I look back on it. It was always getting validation and anything to get attention, but it didn't come from within. I went through my childhood, and I was a very successful little kid in school. I always got straight A's. I always tried hard. In middle school, though, I was an awkward kid. I got bullied a lot because I wanted to get straight A's, but that wasn't cool. It was nerdy and I didn't want to be nerdy.

It was this big struggle for me and it caused me a lot of depression. I would wear sweatpants to school and the popular kids would be using drugs and having boyfriends and having sex and stuff like that and I never even kissed a boy. It was like this foreign thing and I wanted it. I always wanted to be that cool kid in middle school who I never was. It caused a lot of issues like low self-esteem and a lot of depression. I struggled a lot in middle school, but no drugs, no alcohol, no boys. Then I got into high school and that's when more of an addiction started, or you could say that I can identify it as more of an addiction.

That was with relationships; it was always relationships. I've been in relationships my whole adult life, starting in high school. I had a four-year relationship in high school. I came into my own in high school, so I lost a little bit of weight, and I was in the popular crowd. With that, it's interesting because it went from being bullied to bullying people. They say, "Hurt people, hurt people." When I look back, I regret all of that stuff in high school, because it's painful now looking back, knowing that I was that little kid before. I drank every single weekend in high school and smoked weed a lot. It was always to be accepted and to be in the cool kids' crowd. That was very validating for me. I always had a fear of being inadequate or being rejected or failing or anything like that.

That was validation for me if I was the cool kid or got straight A's. I got straight A's in high school. I was in sports; I played water polo and swam. When it came to the outside looking in, I was this perfect student, perfect kid, perfect athlete. I had a perfect family from the outside, but from the inside, it wasn't like that. I had super-low self-esteem. I hated myself and I couldn't identify why. I remember thinking I had a great childhood. Where is this coming from, acting out, and doing these crazy things? I would drive around in my car with my friends. We'd shoulder-tap and get alcohol. We'd even stuff people in the trunk and drive somewhere. I got caught three different times by the cops. I would have gotten arrested, but they called my parents because I was under 18.

One of those times was in a disco. We'd go to a disco every Friday night and we would dress up all crazy, me and my friends. We'd always get alcohol and we drove down to a disco. We got Peppermint Schnapps, of all things. We drove down there and I was driving. My dad loves telling this story. It was hilarious to him and to me now, but it wasn't then. It was horrible. We drove down there. We chugged Peppermint Schnapps in the car before we went in and I was thinking like "Just be fine to drive home after." We chugged Peppermint Schnapps, we got in there, and within half an hour, my friend and I were falling all over the place. The cops grabbed us. I grew up with my dad being a paramedic and he worked all the way up through American Medical Response, the ambulance company. He knew a lot of the cops. This particular cop knew my dad well and so he called him and said, "I have Hayley here. If you don't come and pick her up, I'm taking her to jail."

My dad came. My mom was always the one who was the disciplinarian and my dad was more of the "I'm going to be quiet and let you know that I'm disappointed in you." They

102

came to pick me up and I was laughing and falling all over the place and being all stupid. My dad's like "Where's your car?" I'm like "I don't know." He walked on the beach flats, looking for my car, and it wasn't the "Beep, beep" kind of car. He was in the middle of the night walking around the flats, trying to look for my car, and he finally found it, but he was livid at this point. This is a story he loves telling and I'm like "That's the least of your concerns, but whatever." Just stuff like that. I got suspended in high school for drinking. We skateboarded to the dance from my friend's house, and I don't skateboard, so I fell all over the place.

We got suspended once we got there because we were all dressed the same and one of my friends got caught. I was suspended from school, but the only part that bothered me with that is I ended up being the salutatorian. It was one under the valedictorian, so I got one B in all of high school. When it came to other things, when I was in high school, I knew how to manipulate the system. I don't know that I fully read a textbook the whole time I was there. I knew what I needed to read in order to get straight A's on the tests. My favorite class is my calculus class. I would do the actual work, but I could manipulate the system.

The addiction behaviors, the characteristics of people with addiction, were definitely there. If you would have asked me if I was addicted to alcohol or any drugs at any point in my life, I would have said no. All through high school, I had a boyfriend for four years. I graduated with straight A's, I think it was a 4.125 or something like that. There was no question I was going to go to college. I went to Cal Poly, but I didn't know what that entailed. I wasn't ready to leave my family, and my boyfriend went to the Army, and my friends all went to San Diego State. I didn't know what to anticipate. I didn't fully comprehend what that meant, and when I got there, I ended up getting depressed, and all I would do is study and then I developed an eating disorder. It's so weird looking back, because all of these things go right along with characteristics of addiction, just trying to control things in your life that are outside of yourself in order to feel in control of some sort. For all intents of purposes, it would have been anorexic. I ate 1,000 calories a day and I would work out twice a day and it was obsessive. I didn't drink a drop. I got out of high school and I felt like I'm done with drinking and drugs and whatever else.

I've done Ecstasy a couple times. One time, I got this horrible speed effect. I was doing this thing at my job all night and I was like "Just stop it." This was in high school and I said, "I will never do these drugs." I went to Cal Poly; I was only there for a year because I decided I didn't want to do the major that I had gone there to do, Kinesiology. I wanted to go to medical school and be a doctor. I ended up coming back here to Santa Cruz and I went to Cabrillo to get my general education out of the way. I thought I'll become a paramedic while I'm getting that general education out of the way. I went to paramedic school and became a paramedic. I was 20 when I tried cocaine for the first time and it was like "I have finally found it. This is amazing." I didn't have a dealer. I wasn't connected in any way with that. It was more of a party thing. We'll do it here and do it there. I remember we went to Cancún one time and there was this random dude. We got cocaine from him and we were doing cocaine.

Looking back, it's like "How did we know that that was cocaine? What were we doing?" That reminds me that in high school, we stole a lot. We would take things from stores just for the adrenaline rush. I characterize that with addiction and also getting away with stuff, being rebellious. One time we were in Tijuana and we stole some stupid trinkets, some fish plate or something that we didn't even need. It was just for the rush and we got caught. Thankfully, one of my friends spoke Spanish; otherwise, we would have been in a Tijuana jail. There is a God and God has looked out for me my whole life in these crazy ways. That was the first time I did cocaine more than just party here and there. We drove around and did it all night long, me and a couple of friends of mine.

Fast forward, I had a couple of relationships where I drank for a time; I drank a bottle of wine a night. I was with a guy for four years when I was 20 to 24 and we drank. He was an alcoholic and so I became one at that time. I wouldn't have said that then. I drank a bottle of wine a night and we would get in these crazy arguments. Just nuts—the stuff that you do when you're drinking is absolutely absurd. Mistrusting things and moving out and moving in and chasing people down the streets and just nutty things. Cheating never helps either. It's not me cheating, him cheating. That didn't help.

After that boyfriend, I met my ex-fiancé and we were together for four years. He had a dad who was an alcoholic and drug addict. I sense that he was having an issue with me drinking and so I stopped. That's another thing where I was like "I'm not an alcoholic because I could stop, no big deal." That relationship lasted for four years. We bought a house together and we were engaged to be married. Three months before our wedding, he met a 19-year-old at his bachelor party and left. He came back from his bachelor party and was acting weird. Mind you, the dress was bought, the people were invited, we were getting presents sent to my house, and everything was planned and paid for. When he came back, I asked him what was wrong and he said, "I haven't been happy in two years. I don't want to get married and I don't want to be with you anymore." I was like "What?" It was two weeks later that I found out about the girl. That was hard.

I had become a firefighter shortly before I met him. I was 23 when I got hired. It was four years as a paramedic and then I got hired at 23 and was a firefighter. I turned 24 at the academy. He left and said he's not paying for the house if he's not living there. Our $4,200 mortgage was now all on me and my family because my parents had co-signed with him because I had owned a house before I had a short sale. It was eight months of utter horror for me. It was returning wedding things and it was so painful. I didn't drink. I didn't do drugs. I was adamant about not doing anything, not even taking antidepressants because I was like "I want to feel this and I don't want to mask it with anything."

It's crazy now thinking about that because that's so logical. It's like "Yes, why would you not do that? Why would you want to take anything that's going to make it worse?" That's the logical part. It was a shock to me, then later in life,

I used that as a coping mechanism when before I didn't. That was eight months and it was bad. I lost a ton of weight. I was 120 pounds, which was 20 pounds less than I am now. Everyone at work was worried about me, but I was still working.

Then it was all about guys. I ended up being with a married guy who I work with and again searching for validation outside myself. It was horrible because I was lonely and now I was getting attention from somebody. That then fed this whole low-self-esteem because I felt terrible because I wasn't in line with my morals and values. That caused me to have lower self-esteem, and then we started drinking together.

I ended up having a bad series of calls that we went on, like a bad suicide call in 2015. It was this guy who had slit his throat back and forth in front of the cops. He was up in a three-story window, and he slit his throat back and forth and then he stabbed himself in the chest with the butcher knife over and over again and then fell head-first out this window onto the ground. I had to pronounce this guy. For whatever reason, you take 16 years of doing this and I've seen these horrible things and then this call for some reason strikes this nerve. I started having these horrible nightmares. I started hating my job and not wanting to go to work and having bad anxiety at work. I would get panicked when I would be driving a fire engine to a call that was some suicide call. I would go home and I started drinking in the morning. It was bizarre because I never drink by myself and I never drink in the morning. It was straight vodka. It went from socially drinking to drinking all the time. Fast forward a little before that, I had become suicidal and depressed. This was before the drinking started. I hadn't even started drinking or doing drugs, but I became depressed after this call and I was suicidal.

"These are your options—we can either put you on a hold or we can treat your symptoms and let you go." What was I going to say? I was going to say, "Let me go. Treat my symptoms." I know I needed help, but I didn't want to be put on a 51/50 hold. That's what we do at work. We put people on 51/50 hold and the stigma in my mind was they're crazy because that's what everyone at work says. We want to laugh about it and somehow distance ourselves from it like "We're not crazy. Those people are crazy." It's weird, because every time I've ever had some weird judgment in my head about somebody, it's like "Here you go; you're going to have that now." I ended up being put on a hold. The third time, I went to the hospital because it persisted. That was one of the most humbling experiences I've ever had in my life. I was in the hospital for nine days. They had put me on Prozac before I went in there and that worsened the suicidal ideations. I had a plan like I was just going to drive head-on into a semi. I was driving when my friend called. Goda has intervened so many times in my life. When I look back, I truly am blessed for the series of events that have happened in my life to bring me to this point. My friend called me. I drove to the hospital and met a bunch of my friends there.

My parents were on the phone with me and that was one of the most humbling experiences of my life because for once now I'm on the other side. I'm normally on the side where we put people on 51/50 hold, and now, I'm in the hospital on a 51/50 hold. I learned that they were not crazy there; they're just people who are going through hard times in life. I met some good friends there and I learned a lot. Then I get out, but my coping skill was "I'm going to drink and drink." I drink in the mornings and all day. It did end up being all day long and it got progressively worse. I remember one Halloween, I was with my mom and we were passing out candy because we do that every year. I was falling all over the place and she was like "Hayley, you can't even function, whatsoever." I didn't think much of it because they've seen me like this before, tons of times, but that was in high school. I had this obsession with trying cocaine again. I knew that cocaine was something I liked before. Now I understand why I wanted to try that again because I'm like "It does go along with the alcohol." A guy at work got me the cocaine because that's the only person I knew who I could get it from.

I got some from him and started doing it. I didn't realize before that if I drink and do cocaine, then the cocaine takes away the feeling of being super-drunk. Then people don't know you're drunk or so you think. I got to the point where I was drinking a gallon of vodka every two days and doing an eight ball of cocaine two times a week. It was so much that I ended up getting the dealer's number. I was able to skirt the guy at work and go to the dealer. That was the demise of me right there because then I would just call him all the time. He started coming over and saying, "This isn't all for you, is it?" I'm like, "No, I do it with all of my friends." I did it at my house. All I would do is drink and do cocaine all day at my house, by myself, and literally, no one knew. My parents didn't know; my friends didn't know. I thought if no one knew it wouldn't hurt them. I'm not affecting anybody but myself. I truly didn't think that I did. I wasn't stealing from people. I thought I'm not lying to you if I'm not answering your phone call. I do it all day at work. I was obsessively watching PTSD videos and I ended up writing a proposal for my department to change our behavioral health system.

That was one of the bonuses of doing drugs and drinking, while sitting by yourself and thinking about what your problems are. I ended up getting into another bout of relationships with a married guy at work. It was self-destructive behavior. I remember thinking, "I'm already screwed. I already feel like crap. I already don't want my job. They might as well fire me. I'm worthless and so I might as well screw my life up more." It doesn't make much sense. There is a part giving me validation to be with this married person. It made me feel like such crap in the same sense. I felt horrible about myself, but it's amazing how much texting and talking to someone and hanging out with them will distract you from dealing with your own problems. I had a friend, Paul, who I worked with. He got fired for doing cocaine at work, and I remember being so sad and thinking like "I don't understand how you could do drugs at work." I never thought that would be me ever in a million years. I thought I was so far away from that, but what I've realized over the years is any one of us are so close to being in any one's shoes. You look at a homeless person, and in a second, I could be homeless if I lost my job and then it'd be a chain reaction.

I've realized so much more over the years that it would be a blink of an eye before I would be in anyone else's situation, especially the way my disease progressed over the last two years. It was literally two years, the cocaine and alcohol. I ended up starting to do cocaine at work. I wouldn't drink at work because I knew that that was bad and that would impair me from driving, but I drove great on cocaine. I wouldn't do it when I was driving at work, but I remember before doing that, I had been doing so much when I wasn't working. I came into work and I remember driving to a call, and all of a sudden, my nose started bleeding and I was driving. I got to the call and my captain who was sitting next to me saw my nose bleeding, and I was like "My nose is bleeding." I stopped, I parked, and we were at the call. He goes "You take care of your nosebleed and then come in here." The call was very benign and we ended up getting canceled from it, but I remember them getting back in the engine and they go, "What, too much cocaine?" I'm like "Whatever."

It was a joke; they didn't think that I would ever do cocaine. I know that and the sad thing is I rode on the fact that everyone thought I would never do that stuff. Everyone thought I would never do cocaine. Not that I was perfect in any way. Relationships, they knew that I would pick horrible people. I feel like I have to beat my head against the wall multiple times in order to learn something every single time. I've definitely had to do that with relationships and also drugs. I rode on that, that no one would think I did anything. Another thing that ended up happening when I was using was as it progressively got worse, I was using so much that I would use to a point in the night or in the early morning that if I stopped at that point, I would be able to fall asleep, knowing that I'll wake up in the morning to be able to go to work. If it passes a certain time, I would keep doing it all night because I thought I'm never going to wake up.

One time, I fell asleep. Actually, this happened twice. The first time, I had been talking to this married guy the night before and I was talking to him about 13 Reasons Why, the show on Netflix. I was texting and I was saying, "Watch this show and you'll understand what I've been talking about." I wasn't suicidal, but that show is about suicide in the end. I was talking about all the stuff that she dealt with before that led up to that. When he woke up in the morning and saw that text message, he got freaked out and started calling me while I was sleeping. He called 10 times and I didn't pick up. Other people were calling; I didn't pick up.

They got scared and they sent the cops over to my house. The cops get there, and I'm like "What is going on?" They brought a social worker because they were worried that I committed suicide just because the show is about suicide and I was texting. I have a plate of cocaine on the side of my bed and a bottle of vodka right next to it because that's the way I operated. I'd sit in bed with that on the side of my bed. I answered the door and I'm like "I got to go to the bathroom." I ran and threw all the cocaine under my bed and I'm like "What the heck?" I go out there and the social worker's like "We want to address these text messages that you sent." I'm like "Are you kidding me? Do I have to explain?" Now I have to explain to the cops that I was with a married guy at work and this whole thing happened because of that. This is embarrassing.

Long story short, I was with them for an hour and then they left and I didn't get caught. I've never been arrested. I've never had anything concrete like "This is going to make you learn." I've had to prevent that in a sense like "This is going that way." The second time again, I'd never missed work or anything. I never just didn't show up. One morning I didn't wake up for work, and apparently the cops had knocked on my door, but I didn't hear them. All of a sudden, they're yelling through the window, "Hayley, Hayley," and I'm like "What?" I didn't know that it was a cop who was yelling through my window. I went to the door and there was a cop standing on the side of the window as if I have some weapon or something. There's one at the door and there's one over by my bedroom and I'm like "What is going on?" They're like "Your chief sent us here because we're doing a welfare check. You need to call your chief because you didn't show up at work." I was like "What, I'm supposed to work today? I totally forgot that I was supposed to work." Again, cocaine and vodka in my room and the cops are there and I didn't show up for work. It broke my heart because I went into work and my captain gave me a big hug and he's like "I thought you were dead somewhere. I thought you drove your car off a ditch driving into work. We had people going to look for you, up 17."

I started to realize the impact that my using was having on other people in the sense that they were worried. I was causing other people to be worried about me.

I was piling up bags of garbage outside my house. It's odd because I'm so OCD and clean; that it's the opposite of me. These bags of garbage are piling up on the outside of my house. It was this big pile of white bags and my house is on a corner; it's on display. Anyone who drives by is like "What's going on there in my house?" My car wouldn't move and my blinds are always shut. Ironically, there's another God intervention. I'm writing this proposal for work and my coworker sends me this e-mail about this firefighter rehab place for PTSD and substance abuse. At this point, I'm like "No, I do not have a drug problem or an alcohol problem. I just have a PTSD problem, and once that's fixed, all this other stuff will go away for sure." He sends me this email and it's also before the report or the proposal I'm doing and I end up going. I literally text him back and I'm like "I'm going to call them and I'm going to go," and he's like "What?" because no one knows. I had told people that I was having this PTSD problem or PTSD symptoms. I was having nightmares and it brought back a lot of other calls I had. Every single other call that stuck with me, like hangings in particular. I had this 18-year-old girl hanging that was right when I got hired and then my friend, Nate, had committed suicide when I was just doing the fire service. I'd been there two years, so that was 2008. He hung himself. I particularly had a hard time in hangings and I had another call during this time right before I went off work with this 18-year-old girl.

We showed up and she had an electrical cord around her neck and she was on the other side of the balcony on her deck ready to jump. The cops were trying to distract her and then pull her over the balcony before she jumped off, and it was a three-story balcony. I remember I was able to sit there and talk to her because I had been on a 51/50 hold, and now I was going to have to put her on one. This whole experience had helped me with my job because now I could know what hospital to send her to. I didn't want to send her to Valley Medical Center. I wanted to send her to El Camino Mountain View because that's a better hospital and it will get her the help she needs. When it comes to that, in particular, I was so happy that I was on the call, but then I started having nightmares about it. I couldn't stop thinking about what if she had jumped, then what would we do? I was obsessing about it. It was reminding me of that call I had when I was brand-new and it was this 18-year-old girl who had hung herself. There was those couple of calls and it spiraled inside of me, so I ended up going like "I need to go to this rehab." I called them and they were able to get me in two or three days from that point.

I booked a flight, and dumb me who's thinking I'm going to live it up until I get there, bringing cocaine on the plane. I brought it on the plane with me. I didn't even hide it. I was drinking vodka out of water bottles because that's what I do. I'd drive around with a water bottle full of water and a water bottle full of vodka and a lot of cocaine. I do cocaine in the center console of my car while I'm driving and falling and stupid. I can't believe what a hazard I was for multiple reasons. I end up getting to Denver. It was the connection flight and I missed my connector because I was drinking too much. I had to spend the night at a hotel, which for me was like "Yes, one more night of living it up."

I drank and did cocaine all that night. I stayed up until God knows when. I got on a flight the next day and ended up getting into the rehab and they were joking a ton about "You showed up in this way and that way and messed up," but I don't even remember the first week I was there. I was in detox. I was so shaky and so messed up. I was there for 48 days and the PTSD counselor was absolutely amazing. I still wasn't completely convinced that I was an alcoholic or a drug addict. I thought it probably wasn't a completely normal use of it, but the fire service is its own beast in the sense that when people are working, they can't wait to get off to go drink. It's like "We're not alcoholics, because we don't drink on the two days that we're working, so that that doesn't qualify us to be an alcoholic." I'm like "What are you talking about? You guys drink all day long every day when you're off. How is that not? You know you can't at work."

I got out of rehab and ended up relapsing right away. It almost was like "Screw you to the rehab," because some shady stuff happened when I was there with the administration. It was more of a "Screw you," but I was screwing myself. It wasn't doing any harm to anybody else, but me. In 2017, I was in an IOP (outpatient program) for four months and then I got sent out on a fire.

After that, I started relapsing here and there. I'd have a couple of months and then I'd relapse, and then I'd have a couple of more months and then I'd relapse again. Then it was a month and then it was two weeks. When they talk about progressive, I truly feel that's an understatement. I thought in the beginning when they're talking about that, I'm like "That's a bunch of crap. Progressive? Please, if I don't use or drink and I start again, I'll be fine." Then I got this idea that if I relapse, I'm going to go balls-to-the wall crazy, and that's been my whole life. I feel like everything is balls-to-the-wall nutty."

I know another crazy stupid thing I did when I was using is when they talk about "I tried religion or I tried this or tried that," I do believe in God. I am a Christian and I know a lot of my behaviors aren't in line with that and it makes me feel terrible. I would go to church to try to be doing good and I would be doing lines of cocaine in the bathroom. It doesn't even make any sense because it's an oxymoron or a contradiction. It's me again feeling terrible about myself.

When I got out and I relapsed a few times, I ended up signing back up for IOP. I had a couple of bad relapses and they were around relationships. I remember I got into a three-month relationship with this guy who kept telling me I'm not an addict, like "You're not an addict?" It was like "How long have you known me?" "Why?" "Because I have a good job and a house and I function, but that doesn't mean I'm an addict?"

In his defense, that's what I thought. I would've never been like "That person's an addict or an alcoholic because they were functioning." I never thought my parents were addicts or alcoholics, same thing. They're not addicts; they're more alcoholics, but regardless, I never knew that they were technically qualified as that, because they would drink a number of drinks at night, not a ton, where they're blacking out, but enough to make their behaviors different, and I grew up like that. I've realized now, after a lot of counseling and the rehabs, that a lot of the things that I've done or the ways I've behaved or characteristics of myself have come from seeing that exhibited when I was little and reacting to that. It's not to blame anybody. It's more "Now I can see the patterns of why this probably led me to this or that."

I was talking about relationships. I thought I can try to have relationships, even though they tell me I shouldn't have a relationship for a while in recovery. I'll try it out and see how it is, because it will just go from one addiction to another. I'll now be addicted to this dude, instead of alcohol or cocaine, and that will be a good thing. Every relationship I had that was short, I ended up relapsing after it. I realized fast that's not a good option for me to do the relationship thing. This last relapse I had before I went into Janus of Santa Cruz this last time was bad.

My friend, one, in particular, I relapse with a lot, has a lot of things going on her life. Her marriage is not good and she has a lot of kids, who I adore. Her life is so up and down and she relapses a lot, but I choose to hang out with her. Then I knew that I'm going to put myself around a person who could possibly relapse then I would possibly relapse too, so it's a conscious decision to hang out with someone who does drugs. I don't know if it's this rebellious side of me that's like "I can do it. Even if she relapses, I won't." This last time, we planned it. We were supposed to go to this sober AA camping trip. And she said, "What if we go to Tahoe instead and party?" I'm like "That sounds amazing. Let's get half an ounce of cocaine, perfect, and we'll wait. We'll keep it until we go to Tahoe." We didn't keep it. We got it and we got to try it and then we started doing it. It is an absolutely crazy idea and we thought no one will know. We'll go to Tahoe and we'll do this and we'll not tell anybody. We won't tell our sponsors; we won't tell IOP; we won't tell her husband. We will just go and no one will know. Why do we even think that? Every single time I've relapsed in the past, everybody knows because you stopped calling people and then they get worried about you.

Me and this other friend I speak of, we were trying not to be around anyone, so we had all the blinds shut. We had the door locked, but we had the side door open for my dog to go out. This particular friend comes over—that's my sponsor's other sponsee. She goes around and she knocks on the door and we're hiding in the bedroom because we don't want to answer the door. Tweakers like being ridiculous. She comes around the side of the house, goes in the side door, and without me even knowing it, she's at my bedroom door. She's like "Hayley?" I was cutting up a line on the bed and I looked up and I started crying because I was caught and frankly I didn't want to be doing this anyway right now. This is not fun. She ended up staying there all night. They tried to throw all the vodka our I'm hiding around the house. I hide some in the pillowcase in the spare bedroom. I put a cup in the closet. I put some more in the safe and they threw out whatever they could find. I put the cocaine in the safe, so I was running into my room doing cocaine in the closet, opening the safe, closing the safe, running back out. It was crazy.

That was one of the times, and then the last time was we ended up going camping and my sponsor's other sponsee, my sponsee sister, I guess you can call it, she was with me. It was just her and I. I was doing the cocaine by myself and my other friend, who I got out with, she was doing it by herself. I go out camping with my sponsee sister and I'm using cocaine and I don't think she knows. All of a sudden, we get there and she's like "You're using drugs." I'm like "Yes, I'm using drugs." She's like "I knew it because you keep taking your purse every time you go to the bathroom." I'm like "Whatever, I'm using drugs. What do you want me to say? Get over it." I'm so annoyed at this point because part of me is embarrassed, but it's coming out as just annoyance. I don't want to put someone else in a situation like that, but then she's very controlling and manipulative. It was almost like "I can't deal with you right now, so I'm just going to use." She gets upset with me, and because I'm drinking, for once I tell her how I feel, instead of going along with her plan. She doesn't like that; she gets pissed and she's like "You're just saying this because you're drunk." I'm like "I'm doing cocaine too, so I'm not that drunk." My friend, Jamie, ends up coming up to hang out with me camping because I begged her to come up there and she saw her and me.

My sponsee sister takes the vodka away from me, out of my car, and gives it to my other friend, and I'm like "Hello, she's an alcoholic too. What are you doing?" She drank it, so

I found it in her car under her seat and I'm like "Why do you have my vodka? What is going on here?" Then I lost $500 of the cocaine, but I don't lose that. I keep it super-close to me when I have it. I do it and then I'm like "This is gold here." It's ridiculous, but that's the way I normally operate when I have it. I'm thinking there's no way I could have lost it. My sponsee sister got upset with us because we're doing cocaine and drinking and she wanted to leave. She took my car and she took most of the camping stuff and she left us and we have my friend's two-year-old with us and my lovely dog, Bentley, who is like my baby. We were driving around because now we were out of vodka and we needed more. We're in the sticks and they don't have hard alcohol anywhere. They only have beer. We're like "What the heck; we need our alcohol," and they're like "It will be an hour." We're like "That's fine—we'll go." We drive to get it with my dog and her two-year-old.

If we would have crashed or something would have happened, I hope I would have died because the trauma that would have ensued from losing her two-year-old or my dog or her would have killed me. Just the decisions are freaking horrible. We think my sponsee sister had taken the cocaine, and I said, "Why did you take it?" She lost her mind at me saying such hurtful stuff via text message. I was bawling my eyes out because it was so hard to hear "You druggie bitch and you this and that." I wasn't even saying anything to her. I was like "Can you please drop my car off at my house?" It was hard. She might have been using it, to be honest with you, but I don't know and I can't prove it, the way she reacted. I ended up going home with my friend and we continued to use. My friend's drug dealer came over and he brought more cocaine; he also brought mushrooms. I hadn't done mushrooms in forever, so I was sitting there going, "I'll try some." I tried some, and I wasn't feeling it, so I took more. I wasn't feeling it, so I took more. I wasn't feeling it, I took even more. I was having issues for three days. It was bad. It got me in this bad depression. I ended up taking a bunch of Tramadol also because I ended up thinking I don't want to feel like this.

We were drinking wine because my friend had lost her keys and then I lost my keys, so we couldn't get in any of our cars. We couldn't go anywhere to get vodka. Thankfully, we didn't drive, but I took mushrooms. I took Tramadol, and I was then looking for heroin and I've never done heroin before. I'm like "What are you doing?" I was texting her drug dealer like "Do you have heroin?" Thankfully, he didn't. My next thought was I need to go to rehab and I'm thankful that I ended up making my decision because she was saying, "No, don't go. You don't need to go to rehab. You just get sober with me here. No big deal. We'll be fine." I was like "No way. I feel so bad." I went from normal to completely incapacitated in five days. That's why I say progressive is an understatement. I couldn't function and I love my life sober and everything that I've had and everything that I've worked for, I love it. I truly love it. How do you get to the place where you don't want to even live anymore because of the drugs you've done for five days? It's just beyond me. I never want to touch them again, ever. It's horrible.

What do you think works in recovery?

A lot of things—there are a lot of things I did last time; there are things that I know that I didn't do and I'm doing this time. I would go to meetings and I got a sponsor and I started working the steps, but every time I'd relapse, I'd have to go back. I worked steps one through three probably four times. I would go to meetings, but I'd be so fearful that I didn't want to talk. I didn't want to be seen. I didn't have the confidence to go up to new people and ask for their numbers. One of the hindrances I had was I had friends who had eight to 10 years. When I got out of my rehab the last time, that's who I went to meetings with. I used it as a crutch to not go meet other people and get newcomers' numbers. This time around, I'm blessed that I did relapse, even though it's a bad thing to have happened. That then allowed me to meet people who are new in recovery and getting out and doing what I need to be doing. Going to meetings and talking and getting a sponsor and doing the steps and everything that we need to be doing and living in a sober living environment—I never thought I'd make this decision to live here. Other people are shocked that I made this decision, but I truly want it this time. I had to make some changes that I didn't choose to do last time.

What does your future look like, Hayley?

Super-bright—I have so many more goals and aspirations. I want to go back to school and become a counselor and do PTSD counseling for my department. That's one of the areas in the fire service that's lacking and needs a lot of attention. I want to do that. I also want to get into something with recovery in a different way, and just helping people, not for money or anything, but like you do. I love this. I want to have a family. I want to have children, and one of the main driving forces for me with this is, to be honest with you, is not even not drinking or doing drugs; it's finding out what I like and who I am and getting right with myself, so I can choose healthy people in my life, like a healthy guy. You attract what you feel about yourself. If you feel shitty about yourself, you're going to attract someone who's shitty to you.

Hayley, thank you for this interview and for sharing your story. To all our readers, we wish you to stay sober and be happy. Thank you again, Hayley.

My pleasure.

Chapter 7: Drugs Most Commonly Used, Illicit and Medically Assisted Treatment

While the range of chemical dependencies clients can be afflicted with can be extremely broad, in our experience at Gault House, a very noticeable pattern has emerged in terms of the most common substances new clients self-identify as their drug (or drugs) of choice. By far, alcohol is the most problematic substance for the majority of our clients, followed by heroin specifically and other opiates more generally. This is then followed by methamphetamine, cocaine, and other stimulants, and then prescription drug abuse, particularly benzodiazepines such as Valium or Xanax.

Finally, while often considered by many to be relatively harmless, cannabis is often mentioned as being problematic for clients, even if only as a slippery slope back toward their primary drug of choice.

I will briefly look at each category of drug class and the potential risks posed to people in recovery, both in terms of the withdrawal process, as well as overdose following a relapse.

I will also examine some of the more recent treatment options available that "fight fire with fire" by harnessing safer or less abuse-prone drugs in different types of medically assisted treatment ("MAT") that are often considered the "gold standard" by many treatment professionals today.

Illicit Drugs Most Commonly Used

1. Alcohol

Perhaps the oldest intoxicant known to humanity, alcohol is found in all societies. It is because of its universal accessibility as well as social acceptability that make alcohol a particularly difficult drug for many people to quit. Alcohol is one of only a small number of substances in which the withdrawal syndrome can kill the dependent individual without careful management, depending on the extent of their drinking.

Alcohol is also one of the most harmful substances for society at large, with it implicated in a massive proportion of traffic fatalities, domestic assaults, and other forms of recklessness and violence. At least half of our clients cite alcohol as either their primary or secondary drug of choice and many of them have a history of DUIs and domestic violence charges or worse to back that up.

One young man, a remarkably intelligent and capable person, lived here while awaiting sentencing from his court date. Twice, he had gotten into an accident, while driving drunk, which killed his long-time girlfriend, who was similarly intoxicated. He's now doing seven years for vehicular manslaughter, a totally avoidable outcome, which saw so many different lives shattered following a series of tragic decisions.

2. Opiates (Heroin)

Coming in a close second behind alcohol, would be clients citing heroin as their drug of choice. In many cases, this addiction was precipitated by an overprescribed abundance of powerful opiates such as Oxycontin, although the availability and relatively inexpensive cost of heroin has seen many turn immediately toward illegal opiates without first being primed by a legitimate injury or diverted supply of prescription opioids.

The most notable and infamous aspect surrounding heroin addiction is likely the severe physical withdrawal syndrome that compels sufferers to continue using out of fear of "dope sickness;" which will drive addicts to shoplifting, prostitution, and numerous other crimes of desperation.

Another main concern surrounding heroin is the risk of overdose, which in recent years has claimed hundreds of thousands of lives across the country. This is largely thanks to unscrupulous dealers who have cut their products with the cheap but highly potent opioid, Fentanyl, and its various derivatives, which are legally manufactured in large laboratories in China and then smuggled illegally into the United States.

These compounds can be active in microgram quantities, making safely dosing them nearly impossible, particularly when handled by multiple careless and ignorant dealers. Fentanyl has also been found in counterfeit tablets of prescription opioids, which are falsely considered to be safer than heroin because the potency is supposed to be known. Around half of our heroin clients have had at least one overdose that resulted in hospitalization.

3. Stimulants (Methamphetamine and Cocaine)

Stimulants, primarily methamphetamine, but also cocaine, are the next most commonly cited drugs by our clients. Interestingly, while stimulants are the primary drug of choice by only about 10 percent of our clients, they are the secondary drug of choice by about 50 percent our clients, often used with alcohol or combined together with heroin for a shot known colloquially as a "speedball" (cocaine) or "goofball" (methamphetamine).

Methamphetamine has begun to see a popular resurgence over the last few years as Mexican drug-trafficking organizations have taken over production following domestic crackdowns limiting precursor availability and thus shuttering smaller "mom-and-pop" labs. This has had the unintended consequence of driving purity up and prices way down, so where a gram once cost $100, now it can be found for $20.

Stimulants don't have a physical withdrawal syndrome, like alcohol or opiates do, but they do have psychological effects, which are concerning in their own right. After a period of sustained usage, coupled with chronic sleep deprivation, a state known as amphetamine psychosis can develop. This is characterized by visual and auditory hallucinations, feelings of extreme paranoia and persecution, and general unpredictability and predilection toward violence. It is clinically indistinguishable from paranoid schizophrenia (aside from any obvious external signs of drug use). While it usually resolves itself, following the cessation of drug use, amphetamine psychosis sometimes requires the prescription of anti-psychotic medications and a lengthy recovery period.

4. Prescription Medications (Opiates, Stimulants, and Benzodiazepines)

Speaking of prescribed medications, the next most common dependency we see at Gault House is prescribed drugs. These can take the forms of drug classes already mentioned (opiates like Vicodin, Oxycontin, or Dilaudid or stimulants like Adderall, Ritalin, or Desoxyn), but of primary concern to us is the prescribed medication, benzodiazepines.

These anti-anxiety medications are overprescribed to a shocking degree, and it seems many physicians don't appreciate the danger these drugs pose, particularly once dependence develops. Benzodiazepines and alcohol are the two drugs most likely to cause death from withdrawal if not properly managed by slow titration (barbiturates, sedatives, and sleep-inducing drugs must also be titrated down).

The post-acute phase of withdrawal can be especially miserable, which makes adherence to a long-term commitment to recovery much more difficult. Benzodiazepines have been implicated in numerous overdose deaths; and while few people cite them as their primary drug of choice, they are extremely popular in combination with other drugs, such as opiates and stimulants. The risk of opioid overdose rises dramatically when "benzos" are in the mix. Furthermore, these drugs have been used in numerous cases of sexual assault because they have a tendency to cause a total loss of memory.

Regardless of which prescription drug or drugs a person might be struggling with, it can often be difficult to get them to acknowledge the extent of their dependency or that they even have a problem in the first place. Like alcohol, drugs are very socially acceptable especially when legitimately prescribed by a doctor. Prescription drugs can lull people into a false sense of safety and security around their usage. But make no mistake these drugs can be just as dangerous and ruinous to one's life and relationships as any illegal drug.

5. Cannabis (Marijuana or Weed)

Finally, the last drug of abuse most commonly encountered at Gault House and the one with an even more socially acceptable pattern of use than even prescription drugs is cannabis (marijuana or weed). Particularly as our society moves away from the criminal restrictions placed on it in prior decades, and as selective breeding of marijuana plants and new growing techniques create strains and concentrated forms of the drug that have significantly more THC present, the opportunity for widespread and problematic use and abuse has arrived. Relative to drugs such as heroin or stimulants such as methamphetamine, the potential harm of cannabis may appear minimal, though for certain users, it can be just as addictive.

It is important to dispel with the notion that cannabis is non-addictive. It might not have the same sorts of physical withdrawal symptoms of some of these other drugs, but it absolutely can give rise to profound psychological dependency, especially with some extracts containing more than 90 percent THC. Cannabis can also precipitate psychological disorders like schizophrenia in certain populations as well as a recently identified disorder known as cannabinoid hyperemesis syndrome that causes severe and uncontrollable vomiting.

Cannabis has some clinical use, and for many regular folk, cannabis may never cause them any issues, but the same can be said for alcohol or even stronger drugs of abuse. For the percentage of the population that is prone to chemical dependency, the only proven solution is total abstinence. In a sober living setting, one of the biggest detriments that cannabis poses to a client is its deceptively benign nature—"Well, at least it's not their drug of choice." And then very rapidly they find themselves unable to manage their use or they return to their drug of choice, for which cannabis had been acting as a surrogate, and then their life has spiraled out of control once again.

Medically Assisted Treatment (MAT) Drugs Most Commonly Used

In recent years, a number of treatment for certain forms of chemical dependency have been developed that have greatly improved a person's chances at attaining sustained recovery particularly around opioid addiction.

1. Methadone and Suboxone

Methadone was introduction in the 1970s and then the more recent and widely accessible options of Subutex and Suboxone (both trade names for buprenorphine). Addicts, especially those with a history of numerous relapses, have a range of choices to help support their chances at maintaining sobriety. At Gault House, we see many more clients on methadone and Suboxone than any other forms of medically assisted treatment and they are often considered to result in the most successful outcomes overall.

Personally, I encourage Suboxone over methadone for a few reasons. On a pharmacological level, buprenorphine is a mixed agonist-antagonist that provides both a blocking effect to discourage relapse as well as a ceiling effect that makes abusing the medication itself very difficult. It also contains a small dose of Naloxone to discourage any attempts at abuse.

On the other hand, methadone is a pure agonist, similar to heroin, and this allows the client the opportunity to use other opiates on top of their methadone and provides more of a "high" that is lacking in someone treated with buprenorphine-based medications.

Practically speaking, the antiquated policies governing how methadone can be provided to clients makes using it potentially troublesome. Clients must go to a clinic to receive their dosage of the medication on a daily basis until they build up a trust level over a lengthy period of time to earn "take-home" doses. This by itself wouldn't necessarily be a terrible model; however, many folks who hang out around the clinics are not committed to recovery, or are still using drugs in conjunction with their methadone, and this environment can present a risky situation for someone who is trying to abstain from all other drugs of abuse. It also makes scheduling a work or school routine potentially difficult, as they have to visit the clinic every day to keep the dose stable in their blood and it can be embarrassing for some to be seen nearby the clinic and obviously using their services.

While the general stereotype of the heroin or opiate addict might be a grungy Kurt Cobain-esq homeless person, the reality is opiate addicts run the gamut of everyone, from doctors, attorneys, and schoolteachers, to construction workers, politicians, and housewives. Protecting each person's anonymity is important, especially as they are now doing the right thing and receiving treatment, and the potential exposure risked by frequenting the methadone clinic may not be worth the reward when there are newer and potentially more effective alternatives available.

With Suboxone, the client can receive the medication via a prescription from their primary doctor, as long as their doctor has undergone a brief training and certification on the drug. As the rates of addiction and overdose have skyrocketed across the country in recent years, some of these restrictions on physicians have been lifted so as to try and bring more people into the sort of oversight and stability the doctor's care and medication can provide. Suboxone can then be obtained from a regular pharmacy, which makes it much cheaper and less stigmatizing for many people. Once the patient's dose has stabilized, it is virtually impossible to outwardly notice they are taking it.

It is important to note that in either methadone or buprenorphine (Suboxone) case, they are still opioid medications that cause physical dependency. This is an area of controversy, as some folk consider methadone to be more difficult to get off than heroin. Also, methadone seems to cause constipation and weight gain.

Unlike heroin, if the patient is ready to come off the drug, it is much simpler to slowly titrate the dosage down to avoid as much physical discomfort as possible.

The abstinence rates of those treated with medically assisted treatment compared to those who did it "cold turkey" speak is significantly higher and any available treatment that will help turn the tide of overdose deaths is a welcome addition to our collective toolkit.

While less common, in our experience at Gault House, there are a handful of other therapies available to assist in recovery.

2. Vivitrol

Vivitrol has been introduced to the market in the last 10 years. It is an injection of the opioid agonist naltrexone that gets slowly released into the bloodstream over the course of a month. Its goal is to completely block the effects of any opiates if the person were to attempt to relapse. Interestingly, it has also been used (along with an oral form) to treat alcoholism, as it apparently removes any of the pleasurable sensations from alcohol. The danger here is the person may attempt to drink or use far more than they normally would in pursuit of a high, and this could inadvertently result in alcohol poisoning or an overdose.

3. Antabuse

The drug Antabuse blocks an enzyme in the liver that breaks down alcohol so that if a patient drinks alcohol while taking it, they become violently ill, and as the theory goes, won't drink again, due to the unpleasantness of their prior experience. However, this is easily circumvented by the person simply stopping taking the medication before they begin drinking again; at least, in this case, the relapse would have to be very intentional and preplanned and offers an opportunity to rethink before ultimately deciding to start drinking again.

4. Klonopin

Klonopin is sometimes also prescribed to our clients; however, it is a benzodiazepine, and while is lacks many of the dangers that benzos such as Xanax provide, it can still cause dependency or be abused. But for those prone to seizures or coming off of very long-term benzo addiction, it is a stabilizing alternative that is overall less dangerous.

5. Clonidine, Trazodone, and Gabapentin

We also get a number of clients who arrive with their detox meds after their time in treatment. These include clonidine (a blood pressure medication that can minimize opioid withdrawals), trazodone (an antidepressant that is used to help normalize sleeping patterns disrupted by withdrawal from most drugs), and Gabapentin, also known as Neurontin, a drug originally used to treat things like fibromyalgia and nerve pain, but has since been prescribed widely off-label for numerous conditions. Gabapentin seems to reduce the severity of opioid withdrawal and may also have a calming anti-anxiety effect. The best part of all three of these medications is they aren't able to be abused and are safe among a population who might be inclined to misuse their meds.

6. Ibogaine

One of the most interesting treatments on the horizon that is currently being explored is Ibogaine, which is a Schedule I psychedelic drug derived from the root of a bush native to West Africa. While it is not currently known exactly how the compound has a therapeutic effect, it appears to have a remarkable and almost immediate impact on eliminating opioid withdrawal. Although the physical symptoms of withdrawal can generally last anywhere from one to three weeks, if a dose of Ibogaine is taken just as a patient is entering the beginning stages, it seems to halt the effects and block them for the duration, as well as eliminate the post-acute withdrawal phase for a couple of months afterwards.

Some have described it as an "off switch" for heroin addiction and say the dreamlike nature of the psychedelic experience provides a therapeutic space to help work through some of the personal issues or traumas that might have been keeping them stuck in their addiction. More research needs to be done and it remains illegal in the United States, although there are numerous clinics in Mexico, Canada, and elsewhere offering the treatment to desperate clients, and much of the testimonials are promising.

In my opinion, all drug use should be legal and tracked, as this is the best way to control the black market and solve the problems faced by drug addicts.

Aftercare is incredibly important; there are no magic bullets when it comes to addiction. Relapse is almost an unavoidable certainty if the recovering addict returns to their old living situation without continuing care.

The most effective overall solution following detox, whether with or without medically assisted treatment, is moving into a stable supportive sober living environment that can help keep the client safe and hold them accountable for those critical first six months back out into "normal" society.

At a sober living home, they can meet and befriend others recovering addicts who can relate to them on a personal level and these relationships provide camaraderie outside of the previous social circles centered on the addiction.

Case Study: Mike: All Before 18 Years Old

Mike is 25 years old and has been addicted to heroin as well as crystal meth and other drugs. Mike is from Concord, California, and has three months' clean time. Thanks for coming, Mike. How did your addiction get started?

I was about 13 when I tried drinking alcohol and all hell broke loose. I got a bottle of Captain Morgan with my buddy, Mason—it was the big bottle, the gallon. We thought we were cool and we were drinking with these girls, but they weren't drinking. My buddy, Mason, and I killed the whole bottle. We were walking up the street. Next thing, Mason fell and he's got the bottle. It shattered and he fell on it. His hand got all split open and I was drunk. I was like "We can go to my house; my mom can fix anything." I remember lying in bed that night, thinking this is it; I want to feel like this all the time. My mom's door was open and my door was open. Mason was on the couch and he was hammered; he was way drunker than me.

I started drinking heavily after that, socially and at parties. We'd party on the weekends. Probably I was about 16 when I started drinking on weekdays and partying on Tuesdays. I started taking Ecstasy at the age of 16, the pressed pills that fizzle. That was major for my addiction, more than alcohol. You could drink so much more. You feel like you're Superman. Mix it in with some cocaine and it was crazy. The first time I took Ecstasy, we went to downtown

Walnut Creek, and it was me and my buddy, Mike. We were supposed to go to the movies, but ended up taking some Ecstasy and walking around downtown. We brought his cousin along, who was a goody-goody. He never tried drugs before. We were already smoking pot. He came with us. That kid had the best night of his life. I doubt he had a better night since. Everyone was doing it. Before I did Ecstasy, I was against it. My mom told me that if I did one pill I would die. I remember seeing all my friends on it and I was like "They're not dead."

That's what started it. I was taking about seven pills a night, drinking my brains away. I was rapidly taking pills. I got expelled from high school three months before graduation. Me and my buddy, Mac, I would meet up with him on a Thursday and we'd call it the Thursday-night hype. We'd take a bunch of Ecstasy, all throughout the weekend, go to parties, and hang out with girls. We'd be raging until Sunday. We wouldn't sleep the whole time. I felt more comfortable talking to people. It brought me out of my shell. I used to get picked on a lot in middle school. I was scared of who I was. The Ecstasy broadened your horizons.

To me, it sounds similar to my own story. That progression, especially once you started taking Ecstasy, you immersed yourself into the drug culture surrounding it. Back in my day, it was raves and stuff like that. I wonder if you did things like that. For a lot of addicts, we have good times initially, and that's why we start using drugs. There's a big turning point. It gets progressively worse and worse. I'm wondering what that progression was for you.

I tried the whole rave scene. I went to EPR in the city on Wednesday nights in San Francisco. My first time there was horrible. I hate being around that many people. I get bad anxiety. It was cool dancing with girls, but if they're all sweaty, I didn't like it. We'd do house parties and that was enough for me. My friends and I were selling Ecstasy. We were selling cocaine. I made a lot of money in high school. Selling weed cookies at the high school is what got me expelled. I thought I was a gangster and I wasn't. That definitely opened the door to my addiction and to where it led for years of drinking and doing cocaine. And it eventually brought me down.

Norcos definitely stopped me from drinking so much. I quit drinking for a month because I did some dumb stuff to my girlfriend's car. I smashed up her car when she got me annoyed. She wasn't in the car. I started taking Norcos to quit drinking so I could last longer in bed. My friend told me: "Don't take those for longer than 12 days in a row or you'll get addicted." I was like "I'm on day 30 or something," and that's when the withdrawals happened. I progressed to Oxycodone or "Roxys." I used to snort them and like "No, you smoke them." "That's gross. You're a dope fiend." Next thing I was smoking them. I'm all, "No, I don't shoot them. You're a dope fiend," and after that, I progressed to heroin quickly.

What was the cost? Were your friends using heroin at that point?

The Norcos—I was getting scrips of 100 of them for about $200 at first. That was good, and then the price went up to $500. I was spending $500 on a prescription. That was my whole paycheck. And that would be gone in a day. I'd eat the pills by Sunday and I'd get paid Thursday. It was definitely a money thing because I switched to the 30-milligram Roxys and I was getting them for $15 apiece. Now, they're up to $30; that's what definitely got me into heroin. I was smoking 20- to 30-milligram Oxys a day, spending $300. But I would rather go buy some heroin. It's cheaper and it gets me loaded.

What happened after you became addicted to heroin? What did your life look like at that point?

I quit Oxys in August and I went 42 days without Oxys. I thought I was clean. I was only drinking and doing coke. That is considered clean in Concord. I started doing heroin again in October, and I was popping Xanax with it. I remember withdrawing one day and my little brother had heroin and he wouldn't give me any. I convinced him that I'd already done it before. I grabbed the foil. I hit that stuff, coughed through the straw, and that stuff splattered everywhere. He was annoyed. The financial decisions were for sure what got me to heroin. I always told myself I would never do it, and even though I was doing it in the pill form, it's the exact same thing. But the withdrawals, that's what got me scared. I couldn't quit because I was too scared it would kick.

You mentioned the cost of everything and that you had been spending your paycheck on your habit. Was there anything else you were doing to support your habit, legal or illegal?

I was selling Oxys because I was getting them for $15 each. I was selling them for $30. I was smoking away all my profit. I was selling a lot of them and people thought I was making good money, but I wasn't. I was getting un-fronted. I'd have someone in my family or a friend front me the money and I would say, "I was done." I'd go back to the dealer with the intentions of getting done, paying them off, and being like "Quit—but why do that one? You can get fronted again?" I dug myself in that hole many times, and my family and friends started cutting me off. It hurts. I'm in a lot of debt because of drugs. I started selling Xanax. I was copping $1,000 at a time. That's where the real money started coming in. I was smoking that away with heroin. I was getting an eight ball a day by the time I was done using.

What was the turning point that compelled you to get into recovery?

Not only the debt and the feeling waking up every day, but I was also on Xanax, heroin, and meth. It was July 2 and I was up for three days. We went to Waterworld, called Hurricane Bay now, out in Concord. I was blacked out the whole time on Xanax. I don't remember anything. When I got home, I was coming in and out of blackouts. I was trying to go to sleep, and my little brother wouldn't let me go to sleep. I was hallucinating. I was doing weird stuff in my backyard. Pretty sure he said I was naked at one point. My grandpa was probably annoyed. I haven't talked to him about that one. I woke up from a blackout and I went from my bedroom in Concord to my stepdad's house in Walnut Creek. I don't know how I got there still to this day. My mom walked in the door. My sister walked in the door, and she gave me this look that I'll never forget. It was like "I'm sorry." I was like "What is she looking at me like that for?"

My real dad walked in, and I knew if he was there, I messed up. I and my dad haven't had the best relationship. He wasn't around when I was younger. I've always been mad at him for that. I'm mad at myself because I thought I wasn't good enough. I got to tell him to "fuck off"" that night and I laughed. Some people would be like "That's messed up. Is that when you stopped?" No, I went out for another night and I tried taking 15 Xanax, but my friend took them away from me. I'm thankful for that. The next day, I was seeing double of everything. My stepdad said I was digging in his couch talking about spaghetti. When I was seeing double, I called my mom; I was like "I'm ready to go to rehab. I can't do this anymore." I checked myself into detox the next day. I went to therapy for seven days and I thought I was done. I got out for three days and my older brother was on watch for me. I finally got to go home from his house. I went to my house. I met up with my best friend, Matt. We went and got some dope and smoked it. I only got a $20 sack.

The next day, he called me. He said he wants an eight ball but his dealer wasn't answering. So, we had to call mine. I called my plug out in Antioch. We went and got an eight ball. We smoked the whole thing that night. My buddy from detox called me that night. He had relapsed too. He was an alcoholic and he picked me up hammered. We went to the bowling alley by my house. He was buying me shots, and I was like "I haven't been drinking in so long. This stuff's nasty, but I can't say no to the patron." I took a couple shots, and I got hammered off those shots, because I was already high. I ended up driving his Prius back to my house. I left him in the passenger seat and his buddy in the back, and I was like "I've got to go home, guys." He gave me a $20 bill for doing all that, and I was like "I can't take your money." He was like "Take it," so I took it and then went to bed.

I went home, slept, woke up, and I had that $20 bill. I called my buddy. We went and got another sack. My other buddy picked me up from Matt's house and we went and smoked some crystal. I smoked a little too much crystal, trying to balance that heroin out. You can never get that balance right. I don't care how hard you try—there's no such thing. I was up all night. I knew I was going into New Life Addiction Treatment Recovery Center the next day. I was nervous. I called them and I was like "I relapsed, sorry." They were like "It's okay, come on Monday." I went and did 30 days at New Life Addiction Treatment. It wasn't until day 20 that I called my mom. I told her where my stash of heroin was in my room and to throw it away because that whole time I was obsessing over it. I was not taking the program seriously. I was like "I've got all these suckers fooled. I'm going to get out. I'm going to smoke dope. They can go be cleaned—quitters."

When my mom threw away that heroin, a weight was lifted off my shoulders. I felt much better after that. My buddy, Montel, talked me into getting an SLE out here. I never thought I'd make new friends, but the friends I made at New Life Addiction Treatment are my friends for life, people I trust. I love my homies back home and I feel bad for leaving them, but I have to do what's best for me. I made the decision to move out here, and that was the best decision of my life. Now I'm here at Gault House.

It sounds like you knew you needed treatment. Then once you got to treatment you had already set up a relapse by leaving some dope for yourself back home. What was that switch like when you were there and you were "obsessing over it," and then finally surrendered to recovery? You called your mom and told on yourself. I'm curious what that turning point was?

It was the people I met at the treatment center. I knew if I went out and relapsed that there was a chance I could never see these guys again. I wasn't willing to take that risk. I'd even asked before I moved in here if I could go home for a week. The guy at New Life Addiction Treatment who does the alumni staff and gets people into SLEs was like "What's the point?" He called me on my BS because I was going to go get loaded for a week and then come here. Who knows what would have happened? I probably wouldn't have made it.

What's it been like for you since you moved in here?

My life is great now. I know that sounds cliché, but it is. I've accomplished every goal I set out at New Life Addiction Treatment. I got my job back with my company that I work for. I've got 98 days clean now. My mom's proud of me. I got my little brother into rehab and he went to New Life Addiction Treatment. He left two weeks into being there and I found him out here on Pacific Avenue loaded. That was hard. I've gone through my little brother relapsing, my girl relapsing, and my best friend relapsing. Another friend from Concord is out here relapsing, and I've stayed clean through all of those. I couldn't have done that without Narcotics Anonymous, for sure. I'm working a steady program. I got a sponsor. I'm on step four. I'm about to finish up and get onto that step five and get a lot of stuff out. It's going to feel good.

Step four isn't as hard as they say it is.

Once you put the pen to the paper, it's all good.

Other than the 12-Step program, what else do you think works in recovery?

Live one day at a time. Try to think before you do things. Play the right tape in your head. I know I have the right tape and the wrong tape. The wrong tape is me telling myself that I have fun smoking heroin and it's not fun.

What does your future look like from this point, Mike?

I don't know what my future has in store for me, but I know if I keep working my program, it's going to be great. I love it out here. I'm not going back to Concord, that's for sure. I won't last. I plan to run my own grocery store one day, and I will because I've wanted to do that for a long time, and I work in the grocery industry, and hopefully a wife and five boys one day.

It sounds like some good goals. I want to thank you for joining us here and for sharing your story. To all of our readers, we wish you to stay sober and to be happy.

Thank you.

Chapter 8: Family Advice

1. Early Addiction

A question that I have been asked is; "My child is experimenting with marijuana; what should I do?"
I believe this is a common question for parents. There are several actions that I recommend; the first is to engage with your child on their level. Do not use the "my way or the highway" approach. Try to have a meaningful conversation with them about their activities around drugs and the activities of their friends around drugs. Talk to them at length and frequently about this subject. Expose this subject with conversation and do not ignore the subject or allow this subject to build up power or taboo within your home.

If these conversations do not leave you feeling satisfied, a next step is to get the child's agreement that they will consult with a drug counselor either with you in the room or without you present. The younger the child is and the more that the child is using, the more serious the situation is. If you take these steps, you will have more information to assist you to make further decisions, and you will have the input of a professional drug counselor.

In my opinion, sending your child to a treatment center geared toward adolescence for three-to-four weeks is only appropriate AFTER professional outpatient care has clearly failed! Inpatient drug recovery centers cost approximately $1,000 per day and your child may make friends with other people at a treatment center who are a bad influence. In my opinion, it is better to get your child away from drugs and their "friends" who use them. Perhaps they have an interest in sports or arts and they can go to a sports camp or art retreat to break their cycle. Possibly a new school would help, but changing schools has the risk that your child will fall into the "wrong crowd" in the new school and not make friends with any other people. There may be serious problems in the home environment, a parent with an addiction, abuse, mom and dad fighting all the time, lack of acceptance by the parents, etc. If the home life is the root problem, it must be addressed to improve the outcome for the child.

It would be wrong for a parent to think that sending the child away for three to four weeks to a treatment center is going to "fix the problem." The underlying issues that cause your child to want to use drugs will not have been fully addressed; however, the process of addressing these issues may get started during this period at a treatment center.

2. Hardcore Addiction

Another question that I have been asked by a mother and a father is "What can I do if my son or daughter is in hardcore addiction?"

Al-Anon is a part of the Alcoholics Anonymous organization that is designed to assist the family members who are affected by the addiction of a loved one. I have been to many Al-Anon meetings and I find them a source of inspiration to continue running my sober home. It is common for the people who love an addict to break down in tears at these meeting as they talk about the difficulties that they face due to the addiction of their loved one. Witnessing this gives me motivation to continue the difficult work that I do.

In essence, Al-Anon recommends that families create clear boundaries, which the addict is told not to cross, and that the family remain strong in sticking to the consequence, if these boundaries are crossed. In order for the family to HELP THE ADDICT, they must create clear boundaries and stick to the consequences if those boundaries are crossed. For example, the addict may be told he can live with the family as long as he agrees to a daily drug test and he is clean. If he fails a drug test, he has to leave the family property immediately without any financial or physical support from the family.

This is extremely hard for a family to do, so it is much better that the arrangement with the addict be "We will pay for your first month at a sober living home, during which time you must find a job in order to pay your own way, and if the sober house asks you to leave, we will not support you any further." Sober housing is a major benefit to the families of addicts. If the structures within the sober home are upheld, anyone testing dirty for drugs or alcohol will be asked to leave. In some cases this person will be given a second chance, if they agree to a higher level of care.

It is also important that the family is not a BAD EXAMPLE to the addict. It is unfair to the addict to invite him or her home for a celebration event such as a Thanksgiving dinner and half the people who are sitting at the dining table are getting hammered on booze, and the other half is around the back of the house smoking crack. Leading by example is important. People learn with their eyes. What they see other people do, is what they will do themselves.

A wife or a domestic partner of many years is in a particularly difficult situation if their partner's drug addiction or alcoholism is becoming worse, which it almost always will. Do they leave or do they stay? It is important to know, is the drug addict or alcoholic willing to admit that they have a problem with drugs or alcohol? Are they willing to follow the steps in this book and take responsibility for their recovery from addiction? If the addict or alcoholic is willing to admit that they have a problem and that they need help to solve the problem, the process of recovery can begin. It is a long process that takes determined effort and the steps of the process are clearly laid out in the beginning of this book. Without the addict's honest participation, there will be no significant change in their pattern of behavior. The downward spiral of addiction will continue and a partner begging, crying or threatening is wasted energy. If a hardcore addict is forced to choose between a personal relationship and their addiction, they are likely to choose their addiction because they are mentally and physically dependent on that substance and from their point of view, there is no problem. Many addicts will manipulate a partner in order to stay in their addiction and keep the partner happy enough to stay in the relationship. For example, they will say "Yes, I think I should go to counselling for my addiction" but go only a few times and not honestly embrace the journey of recovery.

Professional counselors can help the addict as well as their partner. In my opinion, the partner must be willing to lead by example by stopping their own use of any drugs or alcohol, even if their use is not problematic. If the relationship is going to succeed, the end goal should be complete abstinence for both partners.

3. Enabler

I have met a handful of addicts who have a particular person in their life who is "enabling" their addiction. Most often, it is their mother, but we have had clients whose enablers have been their spouse, a relative, or an adopted parent. Their enabler is giving the addict money that the addict is using to get loaded. Sometimes the addicts are lying to their enabler about the use of the money, but the enabling relationship tends to be a long-term relationship, and I cannot believe that the person giving the money does not know where it is going.

Two male clients, both over 45 years old, stick out in my mind. Neither had ever had a proper job in their life. Their enablers were paying their monthly expenses and giving them extra money when they asked for it. These men are at a disadvantage in that they were never encouraged to get a job at an early age or made to pay their own way earlier in life.

Parents who overly protect their child do not help their child to function well in an environment that is full of struggle.

The parent should not be giving their child everything that the child wants. Sometimes the child has to do things that they don't want to do, like tidy their bedroom or take out the trash. A work ethic should be developed from a young age if the child is going to grow up and survive well as an adult in our current world.

Life as an adult is not easy. There are many struggles and an enabler of a drug addict or alcoholic is funding the addiction lifestyle, causing more problems even if that is not their intentions.

4. Warehousing People

In my opinion, it is advisable for families to seek out a sober living home for their loved ones who are trying to overcome addiction; however, there is some knowledge that the family members should have regarding sober homes.

Today's sober living homes are usually a single-family dwelling, in other words, a building that was designed to be lived in by a single family, not a group of adults struggling to overcome addiction. A single-family dwelling with five bedrooms is a large single-family dwelling. If there were two clients in each bedroom, this large house would only accommodate 10 clients. Financially, these homes are barely profitable. Razor-thin profit margins make it foolish to kick out a paying client, so rules get bend to facilitate a full house. Effectively, this means little or poor management. The result is absent landlords, warehousing of people and "in-mates running the asylum." It is not uncommon for a sober house to have drugs and alcohol being used within the home. If a member of the home is using drugs or alcohol and they do not get asked to leave, they will continue using drugs or alcohol. All the residences of the sober home will know and soon other residents will start using too.

Providing strong management in a sober home is difficult work that comes with little thanks or financial reward. The management staff of sober homes can get burnt out from "parenting delinquent adults" and the standards within the home slip in a downwards direction.

Poorly run sober homes are NOT a good place for anyone who is serious about overcoming addiction. If you are looking for a sober home for your family member, don't expect high quality from the least-expensive sober home. I have seen sober homes advertising beds available at less than the cost of student accommodation. There is no oversight of sobriety at these sober homes. These homes are warehousing addicts and alcoholics.

If you want a good-quality sober home for your loved one who is serious about overcoming addiction, look for the best sober home you can find; it is likely to be on the more-expensive end of the spectrum of sober homes.

A good sober home has many rules and these homes are difficult to run. Screen the management of the sober homes that you are considering and if they are acceptable to you, support the management by following their recommendations. The management of the sober home cannot do the work for the recovering addict. Laws prohibit any counseling of clients within a sober home, but peer-to-peer camaraderie is very helpful. All that the management of a sober home can do is uphold the structure of the sober home so that the addict can live within a structured environment that is free from drugs and alcohol. This environment gives the addict a better chance of achieving recovery from addiction.

Case Study: Blake: Construction Work on Opioids

Blake is 26 years old and his drugs of choice were all forms of opioids. Blake is from Concord, California, and he is 95 days clean. Blake, how are you doing?

I'm doing great. How are you?

Thank you for joining us here. Why don't you start out by talking about how your addiction began?

I have always dabbled in drugs. I have always been curious about drugs and alcohol, growing up in an alcoholic family. I've always seen my dad drinking from as far back as I can remember. I first became curious about alcohol and drugs around the time my parents got divorced. Alcohol appeared to be the stem of all the problems that tore the relationship apart. It caused a lot of issues. I was curious about why someone might choose to drink, regardless of all of the consequences that were apparent. In middle school, I had my first experience with my first beverage. It was a tequila mixer for margaritas and I just drank it lukewarm. I enjoyed how it felt. Me and my buddies drank it, then went out and just partook in some shenanigans. From then on, it was a weekend thing, going out drinking. Then the following year, I tried marijuana for the first time. That one took me a little while. I didn't care for it too much at first. I had to keep on trying it until I did.

In high school, I'd often miss school, as I was always smoking pot. I dabbled in Ecstasy and cocaine and basically anything I could get my hands on. But that was more of a social thing. I definitely enjoyed altering my state of mind and altering how I felt. Before I tried my first hit of marijuana (I remember this very vividly), I was on a bike trail; I used to do a lot of mountain biking, and I remember thinking to myself, I wish there was something I could take that just would make me feel good. I just remember that so clearly. I found opiates in high school. My stepdad had little yellow "Norcos" and I would steal those from him. I remember the first time I took them, thinking back to that time on the bike trail, that's exactly what I had made up in my mind of what the perfect drug for me would be. I continued taking opiates and whatever I could get my hands on in high school. Outside of high school, I joined the Carpenters Union. I was making good money and I would be sore and tired after a long week of working. That's when I moved to Oxys. It completely relieved my aches and pains. It made me content. That was just my favorite way of relaxing after a long hard week of work. Since I was doing hard manual labor, I felt I deserved it.

In high school, had they transferred into using opiates? It's a question I ask everyone. Did you notice the way you used substances, particularly opiates, were different than the way your friends used them? Did you notice the addiction more strongly in yourself?

157

In high school, I didn't notice opiates as a problem. I was taking drugs how I saw other people taking drugs. I didn't notice it as a problem back then. But I always knew that there was the potential for a problem based on my family history with drugs and alcohol. Once I got out of high school, I continued taking opiates, but I took it more for myself; not caring if I was doing it with anyone. And I didn't care what other people thought of me, because I felt like I was keeping it a secret and I didn't see it as much of a problem at the time.

You didn't experience consequences from the use at that point?

No, I didn't take it on an everyday basis to experience withdrawals either. I wasn't fully aware of the ramifications at that point.

What happened once you got into the Oxy and stuff?

I loved it so much that I just continued taking them between the ages of 18 and 21. I took them for a good amount of time, I remember. It was probably about a year. I took them for two consecutive days, consecutive weeks, and months. I remember having a hard time finding them at one point and feeling very sick. That's when I was introduced to heroin. At first, heroin was such a loaded word. When you think heroin, you think of a junkie, a prostitute, someone homeless who would literally sell their souls to get a bag.

That's what a lot of people think when it comes to heroin. I had second thoughts about trying it. What I was told is they would take away my withdrawals. I was like "I'll do it this one time." I remember doing it and realizing this is the same high. What makes this so much worse? At that point, it was how people lie to you about drugs to get you scared away from them. When you finally realize that it's not that extreme, you think everything they're telling you is a lie. That's what I experienced. I continued my use with heroin. At that point, I knew that I was an addict and I didn't care. If something was going to get in my way of using, I didn't want to bring it up or avoid it because I didn't want to stop.

You were still living at home at this point?

Yes, I was living at my father's house.

Did your father have any idea if you're using drugs, especially once you were using dope?

He's always been okay with me drinking since I was young. As long as I got my work done, did what I was supposed to do around the house, it didn't matter. If he knew about the heroin, however, it would not have been okay. As long as everything looked good on the outside, there was no reason for him to sit down and talk with me about it. I was able to get away with avoiding that whole situation by holding a job, paying my bills, and just keeping a clean outside appearance.

You've gotten into heroin and you were still working at the Carpenters Union. What happened next?

I'd been a functioning addict for about a year and a half. When I say "a functioning addict," obviously I have a bunch of problems with that. The way I made my money and my motivation to make my money and to keep working were to get drugs. I was making good money. I have a good stable job. My employers like me. I've always been a fast learner and I have been skilled at my job. As long as I had drugs, I would show up to work and I do a very good job. I would go home and I would run through my checks, spending it on minimal bills and all the rest on drugs. My hustle was a legal hustle of just working and just keeping it together that way.

Did they notice a change in you at work at all? Did they ever catch you nodding out or anything like that?

Work didn't know up until about two years. That was around the time when I was going through drugs way too fast to where if I was dope sick. I wouldn't call into work; I wouldn't show up to work until I got well that day. I would call them and be like "I slept through my alarm, or whatever. They saw a pattern, as every Monday that would happen or close to payday—actually, never on payday, because that's how I was going to get my drugs. They knew something was up and they were like "We're going to have to can you if you keep doing this." I did this a lot. They must have liked me to not do it any sooner. Using heroin and Benzos—that was all

160

I did. I would go home from work and I would get my sack. Me and my girlfriend would use. I remember going on vacations with my girlfriend's family. We'd buy a half ounce to last us not even a week—maybe four or five days, and every time we would run through it, we'd end up having to rush home dope sick to try to get more. That was just the worst feeling. Up until 2017, I wanted help. At that point, I was using heavy opiates. I was using Fentanyl and Xanax. I was using just heavy opiates and they saw them. My mom, she's a recovered alcoholic. She always knew something was there, but she hadn't been in my life at that point. She couldn't say anything to me—2017 was just a constant battle trying to get my life together, get on the straight and narrow, and start mending relationships, trying to live a productive, normal, meaningful life with genuine relationships.

Did you experience, either with yourself or your girlfriend or anyone else around you, an illegal or health repercussion from using? Have you seen an overdose or anything like that?

I've seen a lot of overdoses. Those have shaken me up a lot. The first few times I'd seen some people overdose, I freaked out. I didn't know what to do. The more that I saw, the calmer I would be. People would freak in the background. I'm like "If you're going to freak out, you've got to leave." You've got to check his heartbeat, got to breathe for him, and just keep shooting them with Narcan until they wake up. They'll be okay as long as they have a pulse and as long as you're breathing for them. That was a big major toll, losing friends and seeing all the ODs. I have OD'ed a couple times and it is scary. You don't realize how evil the drug is until you see people overdose or start losing friends. It's an ugly disease. The sad thing is every time I've seen someone OD, immediately after I'm like "It's my turn. That's the dope I want. I want to get on that level." When you OD, you don't know that you OD'ed until someone tells you. Half the time if I see someone OD, I'll have someone videotape it while I and another guy are resuscitating him, just so that way when they come back, you can show them. Half the time they're like "I didn't. Shut up; give me the dope." It's sad.

I definitely can relate to that feeling. When I OD'ed, the last thing I remember is doing the shot and then waking up surrounded by paramedics and firefighters. I'm glad to hear that you had Narcan on hand. Many addicts don't take that extra step of responsibility. There's no point in talking about recovery if addicts don't survive long enough to make it to that point. I'm glad to hear that you had taken that step with it.

All we're using was Fentanyl and that's the devil right there. Especially people who are heavy on the heroin, they think they can handle it. I'd say about 75 percent of the time they OD right there. I've shot someone with Narcan eight times and they just barely woke up. There were some times where I didn't have Narcan. There's this one time, one of my buddies, he was sitting in the passenger seat of my car and I didn't want to give them any Fentanyl. He was dope sick and I was like "If you do it, you're going to take a tiny hit with me." He ended up roping it, taking a fat hit, and I was like "Why did you do that?" He instantly just turned blue and slumped over. It was just me and him in the car. I was trying to pull over. He was turning all blue. I pulled over and checked his heart. I keep breathing the mouth-to-mouth. He didn't have health insurance, so I was avoiding calling 911. I was constantly giving him mouth-to-mouth, keeping my hand on the pulse. I put a sub under his tongue and constantly people were looking at me, calling the cops. I was having to drive to another spot, give him mouth-to-mouth. I was trying to drive to the ER. That's the insanity too. Why should a hospital bill matter to life? I felt like I've seen enough people OD, so I knew what to do. He ended up being okay, but still thinking back on the insanity of that, it's just crazy.

That's hectic, that's super-gnarly, the limits that drugs push us to. In saying that, I was curious what your breaking point was. It sounds like it got pretty bad. What made you decide that enough is enough?

My breaking point was losing every relationship I had. In 2017, I came clean and wanted the help. Once I got dope sick, I didn't want the help. From that point on, I pushed everyone away. I was living out of my car. I started selling drugs and quit my job, which was a good job. Selling dope is easier. Who wants to work in a construction job, living out of a car, trying to find places to shower? My breaking point was just being alone, living out of my car with no true relationships or true friends. Loneliness drove me to insanity and I wanted my family back. I wanted to either repair the relationship with my girlfriend or get the help I needed to move on with my life rather than just covering up all my emotions with drugs. It works for a little bit, but at the end of the day, you still have to deal with all of those emotions. Everything that you buried ends up coming up eventually. Loneliness is the main thing.

Did you ask for help at that point?

I've been in five different residential programs, all in 2017. The first time, I asked for help; the second and third times, I was talked into going. The next two times, I chose to put myself in. This last time, I only told my sister. I didn't want to get anyone's hopes up and then let them down again. I literally almost told no one and I just went by myself. Once I was there, working on myself, that's when I started telling my family, "I'm in rehab." They were shocked that I didn't tell anyone. That last time, I had been doing it for me before I was doing it to make other people happy or in order to get someone back in my life. This last time, I just want to be okay with myself.

What happened with the four times prior to this one? Did you use immediately upon getting out of the program? Why do you think it didn't stick the first times?

I thought that since I'm an opiate addict I'm just physically dependent on it. I don't need to work a program. They were shoving a program down my throat. I was fighting it. I was trying to find my own easier, softer way. In a couple other places, I just left AWOL and then went straight back to using. In other times, it was just like self-will, not going to meetings, not connecting with people. The last two times, I was more open, willing to do whatever it took. This last time, I've haven't had any resistance. I love going to meetings. I've been connecting with people on real levels, talking about real things. Everything was different this last time.

I assume you didn't move into an SLE after the initial time. What did you do differently? You're going to meetings, going to an SLE. Was this last treatment center different than the previous ones or did you always go back to the same rehab?

I went to The Camp Recovery Center in Scotts Valley and I was there in 2017. I loved The Camp. I loved all the people in it. The community out in Santa Cruz is awesome. The last time, I went back to my hometown. I made all these connections in The Camp. I went home and didn't have any social life, as I was too shy to go out and make new friends. I just tried to be a lone soldier and do it myself. This time, I have moved out here and carried those connections that I made in The Camp out here. I'm still continuing to build new ones. A big thing for me was getting out of that hometown, getting out of those constant reminders that if I wanted to, I could get drugs. I was starting in a fresh new city with new relationships and a lot more structure. I'm doing the Kaiser Outpatient program and sticking with that. Everything is new this time. As I went from the first time I went to the program, it was slow. Each facility was like "I need to do this." It's been a long learning process.

What sorts of realizations would you say you've had about yourself and your recovery this last go-around compared to previously?

I have realized that I am an addict. I will always be an addict. The use of drugs is only a symptom. It's mostly my behavior and me wanting to change how I feel because of things that have happened to me and things that I've done in my life. It's realizing that I cannot do this alone. It's realizing how much more out there is to life. There are all of those things and there's so much to recovery. It's like my work in construction. You can work construction for 40 years and always still learn something. It's the same thing with recovery, always learning something. You can always do something different, do something better. As long as you're trying, giving it your all, and being honest, that's all you can ask for.

I believe that everyone has something to offer, whether they have a week in recovery or compared to the person with 10 years. The person with 10 years might have a lot more experience than the newcomer, but there can be

an insight that's just as profound on both sides. What are your hopes for the future from this point?

My hope for the future is to learn from my past and just strive to be a better person. I can still slip up in the future. My hope is to just constantly learn from everyday experiences and to continue building meaningful relationships just to be content with myself. I can struggle with depression and that's okay. It's okay not to feel good every single day. That's not what recovery is about. Recovery isn't being this happy-go-lucky person the rest of your life. It's just learning how to cope with life on life's terms. If you're sad, that's okay. Reach out to someone and talk about it. At the end of the day, that will better your relationship with yourself and with those other people who you share your feelings with. Just family and just experience life, that's all I can ask for.

Do you have any goals with maybe getting back into the trades, some other idea or direction you can go in that part of your life?

As much as I've thought that I've burnt my bridges with my employer, they're still asking for me to come back, which is crazy to me. I still plan on going back to working construction when I'm ready. I'm just taking each day one day at a time. I plan on continuing my carpentry and moving up one day, becoming a supervisor possibly. I might end up going back to school and learn project management or something, maybe start my own company. I'm just taking life as it comes.

It's amazing how many doors open for you when you get off drugs. The possibilities are truly endless. What advice would you have for somebody else who's considering getting into recovery? Maybe they're hesitant or feel trapped in that lifestyle.

If you're considering recovery, give it a shot. If you're not happy with it, you can go out and you can definitely keep doing what you're doing. Hopefully, you'll get another chance to come back and keep trying. What I've learned is there's no shame in coming back to the rooms. It happens to everyone. There are guys who had been sober for 15 years and ended up going out. As long as you keep coming back and giving it a shot, that's all that matters. I feel truly blessed to not be dead. It is definitely worth it. If you don't get it the first time, you've got to jumpstart on the second time. Just try to stay alive.

That was a powerful story. I appreciate you doing this with us. Thanks to all of our readers for joining us, and we wish you to stay sober and be happy.

Thank you.

Chapter 9: Patterns That Occur Often

It is impossible for me to pick addicts out in a crowd by their looks, but most of the patterns listed below will be present with almost every addict:

1. Strong Need to Escape
2. Drug or Alcohol Use Started in Early Teens
3. Abuse and Chaos
4. Little or No Connection to Society
5. Poor Decision-Making
6. Cycle of Addiction

1. Strong Need to Escape

Many addicts have a strong need to escape from their thoughts. A common phrase is that an addict "is not comfortable in their own skin," but a more accurately statement is that an addict has a need to eradicate part of their consciousness or to "get out of their head."

Alcohol or drugs is an escape route for an addict. In the beginning, drugs or alcohol can seem like a miracle cure-all for making pain and self-doubt go away. It seems like a logical solution to your problems. If this solution is providing partial results, it is logical that consuming more drugs or more alcohol will provide a more comprehensive solution, and if this solution worked yesterday, there is no reason to believe it will not work today.

Unfortunately, the underlying problems never get addressed. Tomorrow, the problem is still there, and the addict believes that they know the solution, which is to drink more alcohol or to take more drugs.

A vicious circle gets set up and a downward spiral is put in place. I have two recommendations that may help. The first is to address the underlying problems that cause the addict to want to "get out of their head." This approach requires willingness, work, and effort on the part of the addict to be effective. If the addict is willing to keep a diary and write down details about their difficult issues, this will help them to rationalize and process the issue within their mind. I also recommend the use of professional counselors as well as all the other steps outlined in this book.

Another approach is to recognize that the need to escape or "get out of their head" is inward-looking and is selfish on the part of the addict, even though the reasons that they feel a need to escape are very real. Exposing the addict to people who are in a worse position than they are, such as sick or injured people, incarcerated or disabled people, or homeless and hungry people, may help them to see their problems as smaller and more manageable.

The world is NOT a perfect place. There are many imbalances within the world today, much unfairness, many structural errors. These problems are real, but they cannot be fixed in the immediate future. Whether or not you gain a full understanding of all the different reasons that you are who you are, there comes a time when it is appropriate to accept the "hand that you have been dealt."

I recommend that you recognize the world as it is. What is your reality, today? Plan your best route through this imperfect world without the need to get out of your head. Getting out of your head is a poor solution that hurts you and repeating this poor solution over and over again, day after day, will not give you a different reality tomorrow.

2. Drug or Alcohol Use Started in Early Teens

The most common pattern I have noticed within addicts and alcoholics is drug or alcohol use started at an early age, like early teens. Drinking alcohol is the most common starting point, and I have repeatedly heard clients tell me that they started drinking between 11 and 13 years old. Many clients have said that drinking alcohol turned to smoking weed and then doing other drugs, like cocaine, meth, and heroin, before age 15. This means that many adults with an addiction problem had a drinking problem in middle school and a drug problem in high school.

3. Abuse and Chaos

Many drug addicts and alcoholic have suffered abuse or severe trauma. The abuse can be sexual abuse, physical abuse, or psychological abuse. Not all people who suffer abuse turn into drug addicts, but it is common for a drug addict to have suffered abuse. Perhaps the drugs or alcohol offered some escape from the pain of abuse. After years of not fixing the underlying problem and repeatedly turning to the chemical high for a cure, another person has an addiction problem. There may not be a linear relationship between abuse and drug addiction, but there seems to be some sort of relationship.

Most addicts live in a state of chaos. There is not much structure to their life. Most addicts in recovery welcome structure into their life because there is predictability and security within structure and the chaos of addiction has become unattractive to the recovering addict.

4. Little or No Connection to Society

Most addicts feel little or no connection with the society that they live in or the people around them. "Anonymous within a crowded city" is the new normal as well as "lonely within a crowd." As online connectivity grows, there are less face-to-face connection opportunities. This is a major problem within the world today and it is not likely to go away anytime soon.

Single parents are common. When there is one parent, instead of two, immediately there is 50 percent less "parent" in the life of the child. However, the single parent is often very busy working more than one job to make ends meet, so there is even less parent involvement in the child's life. Just 100 years ago, most children were born into a village, and the village would raise the child. The child had contact with many individuals and a sense of belonging. Now most children are born into a city. Neighbors don't interact with each other much and many children get left at home alone with the TV as company while the parents go to work. These mega-trends are not likely to change in the near future and neither is the problem of addiction.

5. Poor Decision-Making

All addicts have made a series of poor decisions. One small bad decision leads to another small bad decision, and pretty soon there is a very bad decision being made. The very bad decision that is being made may seem logical at the time to the person making the bad decision. Incorrect or poor assumptions can get compounded over time to result in addicts having a widely inaccurate view of themselves or of society.

I highly recommend that all addicts in recovery get a sponsor who's opinion they respect and with whom they will discuss all their decisions. Having a sponsor/mentor can be life-saving for an addict. I highly recommend this simple step.

There are many ways to make a decision: with your head, with your gut, with your heart, and subconsciously while asleep. Ideally, all the ways of making a decision will agree with each other, but if I was to choose only one way to make a decision, it is with my heart. Here is what I mean by this: When you make a decision with your head, you write down or list all the good points about that decision and then list all the bad points about that decision. Basically, you weigh up the good points and the bad points and if the good outweighs the bad, then it is a good decision.

This is analytical in nature. It is a good method for a business to make a decision because there is no emotional consideration in the decision-making process. It is also the most common way that people make decisions, which is not good because people are emotional beings and not businesses.

When you make a decision with your gut, you take some time to think about your stomach and whether this decision is making your stomach feel pleasant or knotted. Your gut sometimes gives you a reaction to an intended decision, but it takes some practice to rely on your gut to make decisions for you. Strong gut reactions should be given high importance.

Another way to make a decision is with your heart. What is your heart telling you about a particular decision? I find this to be my best decision-making method and I find that my heart "speaks to me," as I am falling asleep and waking up.

I make a mental note of what I am thinking about as I am falling asleep, what are my thoughts gravitating toward. Is it positive thoughts about a possible decision or am I thinking of the negatives associated with a possible decision? Allowing my heart to guide me has been an important concept for me. It has allowed me to "swim downstream" and "stop pushing a boulder up a hill."

You are likely to have heard the phase, "I will sleep on it." This is a reference to allowing your subconscious to make a decision for you while you are sleeping. I recommend that you sleep at least one night on all major decisions.

Addicts are people with a poor track record for making

decisions. Improving your decision-making skills is important and getting a sponsor or mentor to assist you is an immediate step that can SAVE YOUR LIFE!

6. Cycle of Addiction

Many addicts go around and around the cycle of addiction. Unfortunately, this is common. An example is an addict goes to a treatment program and gets clean while they are at treatment because all of their possessions are removed when they enter. Thirty days later, they leave the treatment center and they use drugs or alcohol on their first day out! The following day, they use again, and within one week, they are right back where they started, except more heavily into their addiction.

Another version of this story is that someone gets clean, perhaps they have been to a few treatment centers before, but now they no longer have health insurance covering their costs, so they detox on their own. This is very difficult and the addict resolves with sincere and solemn intentions, that they will never use drugs or alcohol again. They live at a sober home for the structure and camaraderie that it offers, they get a job, and they do well for a few months. Suddenly, life seems too complicated, they are working longer hours to get more money, so they don't have time to go to a recovery meeting, a relationship is starting to form with another person, who is not in recovery, at a social event, someone offers them "a beer," which leads to several beers, some cocaine, and a full-blown relapse.

There are many versions of this story, but the end is always the same. The addict is back into the vortex of addiction, spirally around and around, and slowly going down. There is very little that anyone can do to stop this cycle.

The addict is the person who has to take the primary responsibility for stopping this cycle and they are struggling to control themselves. Support and guidance is helpful and it is my hope that this book will help the addict to achieve a meaningful life as he or she recovers from addiction.

Case Study: Whitney: Beautiful, Slim and Addicted to Heroin

Whitney is a very attractive, slim, blonde, blue-eyed white woman, not the typical look associated with severe drug addiction. Whitney had her wisdom teeth removed as a teenager and received Vicodin for the pain. This was her first abuse of opiate drugs, and it led her to heroin and meth. For most of the past five years, Whitney has been homeless, living on the streets of Santa Cruz, California. Her addiction caused her to lose several jobs and to steal from homes and stores, and hardware stores became her specialty. Her boyfriend participated and went behind bars for these crimes, and he got clean in jail. When Whitney saw the improvements in his health, she was inspired to get clean herself. Whitney detoxed alone and now lives at Gault House, a sober living environment, in Santa Cruz, California.

Whitney, welcome.

Thank you.

I'm going to start by asking you how your addiction started?

When I was a little kid, my parents always said they knew from an early age that I was the one who was going to struggle with addiction out of my sisters. I was displaying addictive behavior at a young age. I can remember when it started; I was probably in my teens. I had my wisdom teeth pulled and I was prescribed Vicodin. That's when I had my first taste of addiction or addictive behavior. I took advantage of that prescription. That's when my opiate addiction started. From there, over the years, it slowly progressed and escalated to me shooting heroin and meth. That's where it started.

Where did you go when your addiction started? Where did you go to get your drugs?

I think of the last several years is when my addiction progressed and got worse. My boyfriend and I had some dealers around town, but because we were far in our disease, we lost our jobs. We couldn't hold down a job. We became homeless. We were living on the streets. We resorted to shoplifting. I remember we would go into all the hardware stores in the area and load up with super-expensive tools. It got to the point where all the employees knew who we were, and when we showed up, they were ready for us. They would try and create a barrier from the exit. It got to the point where we would charge through them and run out the door.

We were so desperate to support our addiction. We had no other options and we knew that it was most likely going to result in jail. In your addiction, you don't care. All you care about is getting, using, and figuring out how to get more. That was our world. Our whole day was based around the getting, the using, and then getting the means to get more. It was like a full-time job. It took up all our time. We didn't have time for anything else. That's when I started shutting out my family, shutting out anybody who cared about me, because, in my eyes, they were an obstacle between me and my using. I didn't have time for them anymore. My world became small. I would sell everything I owned, including the shirt off my back, if it meant getting drugs. That's what my world became.

How did you administer the drugs?

In the beginning, when I was first introduced to opiates, I would swallow Vicodin. I would take it orally. As that progressed, it went from orally to I would then snort my drugs. I would smoke my drugs. The last several years, I shot all my drugs. It became whatever I was doing had to be shootable for me to use it. It was the final frontier for me in a way. There's something about the needle that I was equally addicted to just as much as what I was putting in the needle. I remember when we were sick and we didn't have dope, we were scrounging around for anything we thought might resemble drugs and we would shoot it just to put a needle in our arm.

You were homeless with your boyfriend. Being homeless, how did you pay for your drugs?

When we were homeless, that made everything difficult because we had obviously nowhere to go and sleep and recuperate. It was difficult. We went weeks without sleeping. I'm not even exaggerating when I say that. We went weeks without sleeping to the point where we were both in full-blown psychosis. Living on the streets, you are exposed to other horrible things like being dirty or unhygienic and not being able to shower. I still have these spots on my head that are growing back hair because I was so far into psychosis. I would scratch at this spot on my head and then I would end up getting these fungal infections that would take over and I would lose my hair. That was a result of being homeless and being dirty. The getting and using when we were homeless, since we didn't have money, we had to use other things to get drugs, which is when we would hit up the hardware stores. If we knew what our dealer was looking for or wanted, we would go get that. We were putting ourselves in extreme risk making these huge stupid sacrifices for nothing. We would put ourselves in a lot of dangerous situations, at a lot of risk, for essentially nothing.

When you talk about risks and dangerous situations, what do you mean exactly?

Risks—we were in a lot of trouble with the law. We were hanging around a lot of sketchy people. We were stealing from people and a lot of those people would find out or they would catch us in the act. We were constantly putting ourselves in situations like that and many of these situations usually resulted in a bad outcome. We were putting our safety at risk. We were putting our freedom at risk. There were a lot of times where one of us would have to go off and try and make the means to cop dope. The other one would have to wait sick wherever we were in a park, in an alley. A lot of times, I was left alone by myself in usually a sketchy place. I can remember lying there, feeling helpless, scared, not being able to do anything about my situation. It was a scary dark place to be.

What caused you to turn away from drugs?

My addiction progressed so much to the point of where I didn't initially want to get clean. In spite of what I was living in, I was literally living in my own shit, puke, and filth, and I was okay with doing that. That's the crazy, cunning, baffling powerfulness of this disease. I was willing to live in those dire circumstances for my addiction. In the end, I know 100 percent, I would have died. I'm lucky that I'm alive. In the end, we both were living recklessly. We were sharing needles. We ended up getting Hep C. Our situation was getting dire. I call it a blessing in disguise that my boyfriend ended up getting arrested for one of the residential burglaries. He went to jail and I started visiting him once a week. I saw the life coming back in his eyes and he looked healthy. He looked clear. He looked so much happier. I would go and visit him and he would get choked up looking at me. He said, "I hope that you find a way to get clean." He was glad that he was clean and he was encouraging for me to do the same. I lay around for a couple of weeks and shot the rest of my dope. I sat there in misery and I was like "I'm going to try this one more time."

I went through it. I called my mom on Mother's Day. "I'm going to detox," I said. I went through it cold turkey and that was probably the sickest I'd ever been in my life. The worst detox by far. Going through it, it was hard to see the light at the end of the tunnel. I give my higher power all the credit here because there's no way I could have gone through that without the help of something bigger than me. That's exactly what happened. My higher power kept me safe and got me through it until I could get to a point where I could start making decisions for myself. Thinking for myself, take the reins and get into my recovery, which is what I did. I didn't necessarily have to go to treatment, although I'm a big advocate for treatment. I knew that if I did what it takes, anything's possible. I knew that I could get where I wanted to be and I knew that I could do this. It came down to doing what you have to do. For me, that required moving into an SLE straight after detox. It required getting a sponsor, but not getting a sponsor just to say I had a sponsor, but really getting a sponsor, so I could start doing the work and the steps. It required me to take on commitments. It also required me to do things that made me uncomfortable.

Somebody once said something in a meeting that made a lot of sense to me. And I think about it all the time. They said, "If you're not uncomfortable, you're not growing. If you stay in the same place for too long, it becomes your grave." I think about these things all the time. Anytime I don't want to reach out to somebody or I don't want to go to a meeting or I want to isolate or do what I want to do, I think about these things. My life is worth doing what it takes. Now, I do all these things. Even though I don't always want to do them, I know they have to be done. I've seen a lot of people around me go out since I've been clean. It's sad, but I'm at the point where I don't get surprised anymore because most people will go out. The statistics are against us. A small percentage of people stay clean and the difference is because they do what it takes and they do what they have to do. I want to be a part of that 2 percent. I'm doing what's been suggested to me and it's working out so far.

You spoke about going to meetings and getting a sponsor. Are those the keys to your recovery? What are the real keys to your recovery?

I would say those are big keys to my recovery. The biggest thing for me has been, as cliché as this may sound, is getting into the steps and giving them everything I have. That's what I've been doing. I'm on step eight and I'd never made it past three or four. It hasn't been easy. I've had to do things I haven't wanted to do that have made me uncomfortable. But I know that doing them I'm that much stronger and I feel that much better in my recovery.

A lot of people get afraid of the 12 Steps because they correlate it to being a religious program. That's probably the biggest misconception about the Steps, since it is most definitely not a religious program. It's completely a spiritual program. I've always been somebody who's been borderline agnostic, atheist. I haven't been somebody who had an easy time believing in God or something like that. It's not about that. For me, my higher power is an accumulation of many things. It's constantly changing. It's not this one set idea; it's a bunch of different things. Sometimes my higher power is the group of drunks, the fellowship. Sometimes it's the gift of desperation. It's constantly evolving and it's more about for me being willing to believe in something bigger than myself more than defining what that thing is. I'm willing to believe in something bigger. The Steps to me is more a set of principles to live by more than anything else.

What does your future look like for you?

For the first time in a long time, I see that I have a future. I have all these goals, hopes, and dreams that I never even thought were possible. This short amount of time that I've been clean, I've already seen a lot of those things come true. My goals and my dreams have been bigger than I ever thought. I'm uncertain of my future, but I do know that it's full of possibility. I have hope because of this fellowship and program. I know that I'm going to live beyond anything I thought was possible. I'm not exactly sure what is in my future, but I know that I have a future and that it's big. I'm excited to be alive.

I appreciate you sharing your story, Whitney.

Thank you.

To our readers, we wish you to stay sober and happy.

Chapter 10: Personalities

I cannot pick out addicts in a crowd by their looks. Addicts come in all sorts of shapes and sizes, all races, male and female, young and old. We have had as many beautiful young women as clients as we have had tough men with a hard look. We have had as many tall overweight clients as we have had short skinny clients. Addiction does not discriminate on the basis of race, gender, intelligence, or religion.

However, there are some personality traits that appear regularly within addicts. Young people (ages 18 to 25) in recovery from addiction for the first time are more likely to show the negative personality characteristics listed below.

These characteristics are NOT true for all young addicts in recovery. Neither are the positive characteristics that I have grouped with older people recovering from addiction, but there is some truth in the generalization.

These are several personality traits that seem common among young addicts in recovery:

1. Manipulative
2. Delusions of Grandeur
3. Gossip and Finding Fault in Others
4. Lazy, Selfish, and Not Willing to Find a Job

1. Manipulative

Almost ALL addicts are manipulative! They are good a deception, lying, redirecting attention, creating a false impression, and cheating. Most addicts are good at these activities because they have practiced them for a long time. They will not tell you an outrageous lie, because it is too unbelievable. They will mix in enough truth to make their lies believable and leave you feeling confused or uncertain enough to give them the benefit of your doubt.

Addicts are good at being manipulative because they have been doing it since their drug or alcohol use got started, hiding the extent of their use from others and even lying to themselves about their use of drugs and the methods that they have been using to get money for drugs.

2. Delusions of Grandeur

I have noticed delusions of grandeur in many addicts in recovery, especially young addicts in recovery. These delusions of grandeur may be induced from the long-term use of drugs. In my opinion, there is often a big difference between the expectations of the young addict in early recovery and the reality of that person's situation.

I recommend that people live in the real world, not some idealistic version in their mind. A young addict in recovery has got plenty of work ahead of them to stay clean, to get a job, and to repair relationships. Fooling themselves that they are going to bootstrap a major corporation or do something that is world-changing in the near future is delusional, especially if the same person is not able to keep their bedroom clean or get along well with their roommate. The young addict in early recovery should take "one day at a time" and stay clean for that day, do the steps outlined in this book, and keep their life in order, get six months of clean time, and then start thinking about their grand future.

3. Gossip and Finding Fault in Others

This characteristic is not confined to young addicts in early recovery; it seems that most people in recovery like to gossip, especially about other people in recovery. Recovery meetings are major gossip hubs, and some people find their personal identity in talking about other people's lives when they should be focused on leading their own life. I do not recommend getting involved with gossip, and we discourage it at our sober home, especially gossip about the management team. A client who becomes too active in gossip will be given a written warning telling them to stop. If that client does not stop, they will receive three written warnings and be asked to leave.

One of the reasons that Responsible Recovery's sober homes are working homes is that we have found that people who do not get out of the house during the day have very little input into their lives other than from the house. When this is the case, it is not surprising that gossip and finding fault in others becomes a big part of what they talk about, because they have nothing else going on in their life. For some reason, people seem to find fault, rather than find favor.

Not all recovery organizations or professionals working in recovery do things the same way. I want to say a big "THANK YOU" to all the people and organizations that provide support to addicts trying to overcome their addiction regardless of how you do it.

Other people may find it entertaining to gossip here and there, but this gossip should have zero effect on your plans or actions. No one really cares about what you did or said anyway; they are just gossiping because they don't have meaningful plans of action themselves.

I recommend that people have "A THICK SKIN." Don't let gossip effect you; just let it bounce off you. Don't react and don't gossip back. Focus on leading your best life and your "plans of action".

4. Lazy, Selfish, and Not Willing to Find a Job

Laziness is a common trait of young people who are addicts in early recovery. Perhaps their background is one of entitlement or they never had to clean a bedroom, bathroom, or kitchen before. Perhaps they ruled over a tired single mother, developed an addiction, and then found themselves in a sober home at the advice of a treatment center counselor. Clients are required to do 5-10 minutes of cleaning chores every day, but this tends to be "too much" for the "overworked" young addict in early recovery. At our sober home, if you don't do your chores, you will be given a written write-up. If you get three write-ups in 30 days, you are asked to leave.

Many addicts in recovery become lazy about "working at their recovery." They stop going to meeting and they stop calling their sponsor. They don't work a program of recovery and this often leads to a relapse, which normally starts with drinking alcohol or smoking weed and quickly progresses to a catastrophic relapse.

Addicts tend to be selfish. Their need to get high is greater than the need of anything else, certainly greater than the need of the people around them who may be pleading with them to stay sober. Laziness is a form of selfishness. A person feels that they are too tired or too overworked or the system is victimizing them too much and this is the reason they cannot do "X, Y or Z". This lazy, selfish person will not succeed in recovering from addiction because it takes HARD WORK to overcome addiction.

The work is not a secret; as it is listed in this book. The addict has to put in the work and young addicts in recovery for the first time are often too lazy to put in this work. Catastrophic failure or "hitting rock bottom" is often required to get the addict into action.

There is a particular type of laziness that we have experienced many times, an unwillingness to get a paid job. We have had several clients who have refused to get a job. We have had one client who relapsed an hour before he was due to start a job. I do not know if he did it consciously or sub-consciously, but by his actions it is clear that he preferred to be a homeless heroin addict than living in a house, working a job and developing a normal life. Some of the clients who refused to work have pretended that they were looking for work, but in truth they were not actually trying to get a job.

In Santa Cruz, California, it is easy to find an entry-level job. You have to look around and talk to people, but there are plenty of job opportunities for entry-level jobs.

We run our sober home as a working home. If you are not doing 20 hours of paid work per week, you have to leave the house between 10:00 a.m. and 2:00 p.m. Monday through Friday. Paid work is encouraged and paying your own way is encouraged. Paid work gives people structure. Entry-level jobs are a good starting point because there is likely to be a progression upward over time. Addicts in recovery sometimes undervalue the power of structure; some are unwilling to find a job and we ask them to find somewhere else to live.

There are several positive personality characteristics that seem to be more common in addicts in recovery who are over 25 years old and have been around the block a couple of times. I find these characteristics more common in older addicts, but many young addicts in recovery display these positive characteristics too:

5. Ex-Convicts Have Structure
6. Friendly, Adventurous Soul
7. Appreciative to Have a Home
8. Camaraderie toward Other People
9. Proud to Be in Recovery

5. Ex-Convicts Have Structure

We have housed many people who are recovering from addiction and who have recently got out of prison. It is noticeable that Ex-Convicts do well within a structured environment. They don't have problems following the house rules probably because prisons are a very structured environment. That structure is provided by the prison system and the guards, but more importantly, there is a strong structure imposed by the prisoners themselves. Stepping outside of the prisoner-imposed structure can cost you your life. The structure within a sober living environment is easy compared to the structure within a prison.

Ex-convicts are good with structure and they generally have an up-beat attitude because a sober living home is a much better place to be than any prison; however, ex-convicts also tend to have a prison mentally, where they position the sober living management team as the jailers and themselves as the prisoners. We do not want that culture at our sober home. Ex-convicts also have a "no-snitching" attitude, and we want our clients to buy into our mission of being a safe harbor from drugs and alcohol. If a client is using, we want other clients to inform the management, so we can get the person who is using drugs or alcohol off the property as soon as possible.

6. Friendly Adventurous Soul

I have found most addicts in recovery to be friendly, pleasant people. Most addicts in recovery seem to like to be around other people and they are social. Perhaps some addicts in recovery are too agreeable and lack the ability to say "no." However, in general, a friendly disposition is a positive personality characteristic that I have noticed in most addicts in recovery.

Many addicts in recovery are adventurous souls, people who are willing to try something new. I find this an attractive characteristic. People with an adventurous soul are more likely to laugh at life and themselves. These people are fun to be around and make me feel light-hearted about my own troubles and difficulties.

7. Appreciative to Have a Home

Many addicts in recovery are appreciative to have a home. Many of the older addicts in recovery may have spent some time living on the streets or in the bushes. Most addicts in recovery appreciate having a bed to sleep in and a clean bathroom and kitchen, and they show their appreciation by saying "thank you" and doing their chores to contribute to the clean environment. Addicts in recovery who are living in a sober home tend to stay positive in their attitude, and they tend to be thankful for having a decent place to live.

8. Camaraderie toward Other People

There is a supportive camaraderie among addicts in recovery from addiction. People tend to help each other out and share information about meetings and resources. Addicts in recovery have a great deal in common and band together to help each other solve their common problems. This camaraderie is attractive and it is another good reason for an addict in recovery to live in a sober home with other addicts in recovery.

9. Proud to Be in Recovery

Most addicts in recovery are PROUD to be in recovery. They do not hide the fact that they are in recovery, and many addicts in recovery will "fly their colors." I find this attractive, and I have noticed it at recovery events, which tend to be festive with many different cultures.

I respect people who confront their problems, even if they fail in trying to deal with their problems. I do NOT recommend putting your problems front and center on social media, such as Facebook, but to confront your problems is something to be proud of. Many addicts in recovery are not shy to say that they are in recovery from addiction. They don't pretend that they never had a problem with addiction. Many addicts in recovery are proud to be in recovery.

Case Study: Luke: Fighting for Drugs

Luke is a big, strong 19-year-old male. Luke would beat people up for their drugs or their money. He grew up in Northern California, considers Half Moon Bay his home, and is currently living at Gault House SLE in Santa Cruz, California. Luke graduated from high school and is interested in getting a trade. He has been to rehab five times and has 28 days clean. Luke used "strong-arm" tactics to get what he wanted, but now he wants the love and happiness that the recovery lifestyle offers.

How are you doing, Luke?

I'm doing great.

Please tell us how your addiction got started.

I was about 11 years old when I first tried pot. I did it a few times. It never kicked off with me. I never liked it in the beginning. A couple of years went by and I started smoking a lot more with my buddies. I started growing it. It became an everyday thing for years after that. From smoking pot, I started drinking. My dad used to grow pot and he drank a lot. He still does. He's an alcoholic. I started drinking and smoking in a small town, going to parties and playing football. I was a football stud. I played sports and everything seemed acceptable. I was a freshman in high school when I got caught with weed on campus. I got suspended. I got in trouble. I got on probation. My parents sent me to this Beyond Scared Straight program. I ended up walking, going into the Beyond Scared Straight program at Folsom State Prison.

They sent you to this program, but up to that point, did you use the same way that your friends did? Did you notice any difference? Did you use any differently than they did?

In the beginning, they used more than me. That's the funny thing. They would always say "Try to get Luke to smoke because he gets all goofy." I didn't like it. I get paranoid and then eventually I started loving it. From smoking weed, my sister, she started bringing it around me more. She's an alcoholic and an addict too. We wouldn't even go to the school. We would sit around the house and smoke weed and party and whatever comes along with that. We go to parties, hanging out at the house, and get high. It was rough. I was abused as a kid, and my dad worked out of town, so he was never there, and my mom was working full-time. We always had a lot of time on our hands. We took advantage of that and we did stuff that kids shouldn't be doing it that age, vandalizing, smoking weed, getting high, stealing, fighting, whatever it was.

Did your parents allow you to smoke and drink around the house?

In the beginning—they were very against it because I was smoking weed at such a young age, but then I found out that they were growing it. They couldn't keep me from smoking. No matter what the consequence was, I became defiant. They would say, "You're grounded. You're not going to hang out with anybody." I wouldn't even care. I would still go do what I would do. It got so bad where I had no respect for my parents, my sister, family, and friends. It was horrible.

From there, I broke my left arm in football game, diving for a fumble. My arm broke up by the shoulder. I got prescribed Vicodin. My mom let me take it on my own. I would go to school and take three or four of them. I didn't think it was going to do anything. I remember I took them and I went to school the first day that I had got them. I felt amazing. I felt wrapped in a blanket, so comfortable in my own skin. I didn't know what I was doing, but I loved it.

From there, I only had a little bit of Vicodin for probably about a month and I ran through it in 10 days. I ran out of Vicodin and that was it. I went probably about another year without Vicodin or without pills in general. I went back to smoking weed and drinking and partying and doing everything I did, fighting. I had another buddy who was like "I got Oxycontin." I was like "What's that?" He's like "It's like Vicodin, stronger though." I was like "Let me try it." I tried it and it was better than Vicodin. It was amazing. I didn't work at the time. I was only about 16 years old. On a Friday night, I would call him up, borrowing $20 from my mom, which I never paid back. I would go get Oxycontin. I would take them.

I would snort them or whatever I would do with them. I would get high. I would drink on them. I would go to a football game all messed up and I would look a fool. I thought it was funny. I thought it was cool, with everybody looking at me, but in reality, everybody was making fun of me. I was known as the kid who gets messed up all the time. I looked incoherent. I didn't know what i was doing. I had bad grades. My football coach knew what I was doing. It was really bad. Now that I think about it, it was bad. At the time, I thought it was normal. I thought I was fine. I thought everybody thought it was cool and it was acceptable.

While doing all that, I graduated from high school. I don't know how I did that.

Would you say at that point you had exceeded the drug use from within your social circle?

I definitely did. Everybody was still smoking weed and drinking. The cocaine didn't come into play for probably another year. I had a couple buddies who would do the Oxys too, but they weren't doing it like I was. The night of getting high, the next morning, I'm wanting more. I couldn't smoke weed without pills. I couldn't do that. I always needed opiates. I always needed pills, Xanax, whatever it was. I always needed something to slow me down a little bit.

My parents got divorced when I was 17 years old. I moved from that small town up north back to the Bay Area where I'm from. I had weed all over my house and bongs. My dad was upset at my mom. He wanted to sue for full custody.

The only reason he could use was that I'm a drug addict and that I have weed and paraphernalia lying all over the house. He took that and ran with it. He got a lawyer, took pictures of all my bongs, my weed, alcohol, and beer cans, the whole nine yards.

He took them and he showed them to the lawyer. My mom was devastated thinking that she's going to lose my little sister. At the time, she was five years old. I ended up having to go to the rehab, The Camp. At the time, I was using drugs, but I wasn't using drugs like these people in this rehab. I was 17. I was in this rehab. People were telling me about heroin and cocaine, Xanax. I tried pills, but I never did it like that. These people were telling me how they steal their mom's cars and crash them, high on drugs, and going to jail, juvenile hall. That made me want to try drugs even more because I learned about all these new drugs that you could try, Molly/Ecstasy, whatever it was, I did take that program. I was not serious at all and got kicked out on the fifteenth day.

What did you get kicked out for?

For not taking anything seriously, clowning the workers there. I had no care at all. I was so upset at my dad for doing that. I was almost doing it as payback. I get out and go back to my hometown in Half Moon Bay. I'm not even enrolled in school. It's my junior year and I was living with my dad. I couldn't go live with my mom because I didn't say anything about it, but I got into my stepdad. He's this big Mexican dude. I came to the house messed up on drugs and he came at me. He put hands on me and I put my hands on him. I took it to court. I couldn't be around him. My little sister couldn't be around him, and that was while everything was going on with my dad suing my mom for full custody. It looked even worse on my mom with that going on. I couldn't see my mom, my little sister, or my stepdad for about six-to-eight months, so I lived with my dad. I didn't even go to school. I started working construction under the table. I would get my paycheck Friday. We're getting paid weekly. I get my paycheck and go right to the dope dealer.

I started buying the Oxycontin at the beginning, the Blues. I started smoking them. I didn't know you could do that. I was smoking them off tinfoil. It went from there. That was the first time I started feeling the effects of withdrawal. It was when I would use heavily for a whole weekend and go back to work in the hot sun and sweat even more. It's so uncomfortable on my skin. I don't even know how I did it honestly, but I would power through each day and get that paycheck and keep doing it more and more. Eventually, the drugs got so bad, the Oxys, the Xanax. It was all bad. I ended up losing that job because I stopped going. I started selling drugs, whatever I could get my hands on, Xanax, coke, meth, whatever it was. I started selling drugs enough to support my addiction pretty much. I always thought I was big time with $1,000 in my pocket. I would blow it all in the weekend on drugs and be back at square one. It was depressing.

How did you get into heroin at this point once you started feeling the withdrawal effects from Oxy?

That was what it was. I started doing the Oxys and they got so expensive at $30 a pill that I couldn't pay for them anymore. I had a buddy who I would always hang out with. We got high together all the time. We grew up together. He's like "I got pure opium." But it wasn't a pure opium; I found out two weeks after smoking it every day that it was heroin, and I didn't even care at that point. I would justify it by saying, "I'm smoking it. I'm not shooting it. I'm smoking on tinfoil. It's not a big deal," but it really was. From there, I started getting in a lot of fights, beating people up all the time. I didn't even feel human at the time. I was so depressed, but I was always high. I didn't feel depressed. I was a goofball running around, beating people up, doing drugs, stealing, robbing anybody for their drugs or their money. This was a small town and there I was doing all this. My parents started hearing that I was selling meth and selling drugs. Somehow I convinced them that I wasn't, but the whole time I was getting high and doing all this stuff.

Did they notice a change in your behavior?

They definitely did. I would come home all fucked up. I'd tell them I'm smoking weed. They didn't know what to do. They would always call the police and have the police come and think that the police would take me to jail, but I never had anything on me. I was smart. I would always ditch it somewhere or get rid of it or I already used it all. They would say, "You're out of luck. There's nothing we could do." They try and get me to pee in a cup because they want to prove so bad that I was using. The cops can't force you to pee in a cup. From there, I found out where my dealer was getting the heroin because I would buy it from a friend who got it from San Francisco on the streets of the Tenderloin. I started going there every day with him and buying it from the actual dealers, the Hondurans in San Francisco. I started using it every day. It got to the point where I got kicked out of my house for robbing someone of their drugs. They came to my house, crying, a grown man saying, "I need of my drugs back or else I'm going to get killed."

That didn't stop me. I got kicked out of my house. I was homeless for about six months. I've been homeless numerous times, but this time I was homeless for about six months, running around San Francisco. I'm surprised I didn't get killed honestly. There had been numerous times when people have put knives up to my neck. At that time, I'm running around San Francisco. I don't know how to make money or anything. I'm pretty much dirt-broke. I started boosting and not a lot of people know about that. In San Francisco, they've got a marketplace where we sell all kinds of stolen goods. The main things are detergent, soap, pistachios, almonds, anything from Walgreens and CVS, all that, and they will buy it. I learned that I could go to all these stores with a backpack and load them up and go to this marketplace downtown and sell it all. I would have $400, $500 a day, sometimes even more, sometimes less. I would take that money and I would go get high.

I did that for about a year. I've been in the streets for so long my feet would be bleeding. I would be out there in the same clothes for so long I would call my mom and have her come pick me up and save me. She would take me to a detox center. I would detox, get back on Suboxone, and start over. There was a cycle of always doing that. That was repetitive.

I started smoking crack out there. I tried crack for the first time. It took about two months for me to start doing it heavily from the first time I tried it. Heroin went out the door. Crack was $5 for a bag. Heroin is $10 for a bag. I ran with the crack, smoking so much crack, an eight ball a day. I was still doing heroin on the side, but my main priority was crack. I kept doing it every day. I would go to the hospital. There are about five times when I would call the ambulance and have a panic attack or my whole arm and body would go numb because I was smoking so much crack. My heart was going so fast, and I would freak out and go to the hospital.

They'd tell me, "You're going to die if you keep doing this." I'll say, "Yes, I'll stop." I go home, have my mom come pick me up. I'll get about two, three weeks, sometimes a month clean of not doing anything, maybe smoking a little bit of weed. I would think I could go back and do it again. I would go back. My main problem is I lived on the outskirts of San Francisco in another city. You have to go to San Francisco to buy these drugs mostly unless you know someone and I didn't know anybody. I could get heroin, but I couldn't get crack.

I would go out there with some money or make some money boosting. I would get high and I'd run out of crack, but I couldn't go home. The crack was keeping me there. There's a Bart station that could take me right to my house, but the fact is, I would get a lot of crack and I'd get on that Bart station and say, "I'm going home. I need to go home." Halfway on the Bart ride, I'd run out of crack and I would turn right back around and head right back to the city to buy more crack. The crack was keeping me from going home.

Do you smoke on the train?

All the time, in the back, in the front, wherever. I didn't even care what people thought. I did it in front of kids, babies, and the parents wouldn't even know what to say. Smoking a crack pipe right in front of kids on a secluded area on a train.

What happened at that point with your family, with your life? Even if you were forced into treatment, going to detox and stuff, you had a taste of recovery. I'm wondering what it took for you to get to the breaking point around your addiction.

The breaking point, when I was smoking all this crack and getting high, I felt mentally unstable. I felt I didn't even want to live anymore. I had no purpose. I couldn't make anybody happy. My only friends were friends because I was supporting their addiction a lot of the time. I would get them high. Once I ran out of drugs, they would leave. That cycle would keep going. I had no real love at the time, besides my mom. She didn't know what to do with me. After that first rehab, when I was 16 or 17, I ended up going to three other rehabs, maybe four rehabs. I don't even know. I've been to five total, but four other rehabs, being clean for a month, when I get out, and then going right back to using for about six months, and into that cycle. It was insanity. I didn't know what to do.

I knew there are 12-Step meetings. I knew there are intensive outpatient programs. There's outpatient and there's inpatient. There are tools, but I didn't know how to use them and put them to work. When I would use these tools, I still wanted to get high. The drugs still controlled me. I would go to outpatient after I was in rehab. I would go to these meetings and I would do it all, but I would either be high at the meetings or I'd be waiting to get out of the meetings to go get high. During that time, I would make up these lies saying, "I'm going to get on the Bart station. Mom, I need $20 for Bart and for food. I'm going to go across the bay to San Bruno and hang out with my buddy, Rob. I'm coming back at 11:00 p.m.". I wouldn't even go there. I would go straight to the San Francisco Civic Center and I wouldn't go home. I couldn't go home because I was too high on drugs to sit around at home. I didn't know what to do.

At the time, I thought it was normal. Even though I was mentally unstable and I didn't know what to do, I felt scared. I felt I was going to die. If I were to keep going like that, I would die. I've seen all my other friends or acquaintances out there in San Francisco and they were doing the same thing. They had the same problems. They couldn't go home. They were getting high. It made me think it was normal. Even young girls who have good looks and everything, they're on a street corner, prostituting themselves and smoking crack, when they're from a middle-class family.

From there, I got on Suboxone. I would do that same repetitive thing over and over again. I got kicked out of the four rehabs and I gave up. My parents gave up, but they were still letting me live in the house. They were accepting it and letting me walk all over them. I would steal whatever from them to sell or to pawn to get high. I've gotten rid of so many nice things that had value to me and that I loved, the expensive stuff, whatever it is. I eventually had nothing. I probably had about four different pairs of clothes. I got rid of my phone, I got rid of everything. I had nothing. I didn't have a TV in my room. I got rid of my Xbox. I had nothing of value.

At the time, I thought it was normal. I don't even need that. That's how I justify it. I was like "I don't need this. Xbox is bad for you." That's how I would justify it. Sitting around playing video games is bad for you while I was smoking an eight ball of crack a day. I had this one counselor in an outpatient program. His name was Mike. He was a great dude. He wanted to see me succeed. We had similar stories. He was clean for about 30 years. He did the same things I did in San Francisco in the Tenderloin. He did the same whole nine yards. He inspired me to get clean and to do what I wanted, to do what I'm doing now. I never wanted to make that leap of faith and that decision. I kept getting high. I didn't know what to do.

I finally told my mom that I needed to go to rehab; I needed to try one more time. I went to The Camp Recovery Center one more time, and this time, it felt different. I wanted to genuinely be sober. I started feeling how it feels to be happy again, to be successful, to work a job, to make my own money, to not steal for a living, to have friends again, to have love. To have people who love me and want to be around me. I'm now cherishing that and it's amazing. I didn't think I would ever get to that point again. I went to rehab. I did everything I needed to do. I now attend meetings and recovery is great. I would have died if I didn't keep going.

This is my twenty-eighth day clean. I've been clean longer before, but this time I'm serious about being clean. I try to keep myself occupied, go to meetings, hanging out with good people. I try not to do anything that seems foreign to me. It wasn't foreign when I was using, but I'm trying to not do old behaviors.

I live in this sober home and I hang out with good people. I go to meetings and I do everything that happiness is for a recovering addict. My parents love me now. They take care of me with love. If I need a little bit of money, they're willing to give me a little bit of money and let me use it for something that's useful. They trust me to go to their house. They trust me. They can leave me in their car with their purse, wallets, and phones. They used to never be able to do that. I've come a long way and they genuinely care about me. My mom, she still doesn't know if I'm 100 percent going to be sober and if this is going to be it. I don't even know that myself. I have to do it, day by day, and that's what I do. One more day and I've been doing pretty good at that.

I'm so stoked you said that because when I was your age, even a couple years older, when I went to my first program, and in a family group, my mom had said the same. She was very upset and said, "Are you done?" I said, "I don't know," in front of a big group. People are disappointed. She was disappointed, but all I could be was honest. I ended up not being done, but your story, especially for a 19-year-old, it's very similar to mine, but in a much shorter period of time. To see your progression and how rapidly you progressed from smoking pot and drinking to the pills to the opiates to the stimulants, but then to also have that perspective right now, I hope that you stick it out, because you've got a good grasp of recovery for having 28 days. Now I'm curious what your hopes are for the future.

I'm only 19, but my hopes are to own my own house one day; have a beautiful wife, and even though I'm young,. I would like to have a job, where I can come home and I don't have to worry about bills. I don't have to worry about how I'm going to survive, whether I'm getting high or not, knowing that I'm making enough money to support me or my family, if I have one. That is what I want. I want to live in a nice area. I want to be able to take care of myself and not rely on anybody. Even when I was using, I was a very independent person. Whether or not I was stealing to get my money, I could always support myself. This time, I want to support myself the right way. I want to have good relationships with everybody and live that American dream life.

People think of America and they think it's all nice and amazing. It's cookies and cream, but it's not. California, there are so many people getting high and using drugs and addicts. It's nuts. It's honestly bizarre. I never thought I would be in that position, be in those shoes. I would always look down on those people in a way when I was young, "Look at that dude. He's a heroin addict. He's popping pills. He is a jackass. He doesn't know what he's doing. He's a fool." Before I knew it, in a span of six years or something, I was that dude. I would never think that I would be there.

My hopes are I'm going to get into the trades, sheet metal preferably, but whatever job comes my way, electrician, plumbing, HVAC, whatever it is, whatever makes good money. They all make good money. I need to move on with my life. Even though I'm only 28 days clean, I need to forget about the past. It's still a part of me. I'm still going to use it to help people and to help myself and be of service. I need to move on and be the person I am and make my family proud because I come from generally a pretty good family.

I was abused as a kid. My mom did the best she could. It was rocky, but it was nice. I try and look at the good things and the bad things that make me who I am. I want to critique all those bad things that me and my family had been though and make sure my kids never have that problem. They don't have to worry about food. We are a middle-class family, but there were times when we had no food in the house. A 14-year-old kid had to go steal food from a market to feed his sister and to feed himself because his parents weren't home.

They were out doing their own thing. There was no food in the house and I needed to eat. I don't want to have to ever worry about that again or my future kids or wife.

I want to be stable. I want to be successful. I want to be happy. That's the main thing, being happy.

I've always believed that we build character through adversity. It certainly sounds like you faced plenty of that. What advice would you have for somebody who's maybe considering getting into recovery and has dealt with similar situations and addictions, as you have?

Keep going to those meetings. Keep doing it. Keep craving recovery. If you have five more runs in you or if you have one more run, keep trying to do better, whether it be recovery, being sober, how many days you have. It's a day-by-day thing. One day at a time. I'm being nice to people, doing courteous things. Try and build your character in a good way. That's the only thing I could say, work on yourself mentally and physically and be a good person.

It's not hard to be a good person now that I'm clean. I don't have to do those horrible things I used to do to get what I need. It doesn't take a lot of time out of your day to help someone with anything. Help an elderly person with their groceries, help a friend, give him a ride, whatever it is. Buy a homeless person some food. Keep trying to better yourself in that way where you make yourself happy, you feel of service, and that gives that person one more chance, a chance at life again, whether it's someone homeless or someone in the struggle or someone who needs help. Work on yourself.

I appreciate you sharing your story with us. To all our readers, we wish you to stay sober and be happy.

Chapter 11: The Benefits of Being Clean and Sober

There are many benefits of being clean and sober:

1. Lower Risk of Incarceration
2. Lower Risk of Injury and Disease
3. Lower Risk of Death
4. More Conscious and More Fun
5. More Power and More Respect
6. Consistent Thought Patterns
7. Better Relationships
8. More Meaningful Life

1. Lower Risk of Incarceration

The Federal Bureau of Prisons reports that approximately 46 percent of all inmates are in prison for drug offenses, by far the highest reason for incarceration. Weapons, explosives, and arson account for the next 20 percent of inmates and sex offenders are the third-highest number of prisoners, with 10 percent of inmates. The remaining 24 percent of inmates accounts for crimes related to banking and insurance, counterfeit and embezzlement, burglary, larceny, property offenses, continuing criminal enterprises, extortion, fraud, bribery, homicide, assault, kidnapping, immigration, national security, and robbery. It is amazing that all these offenses combined account for approximately half the number of prisoners doing time for drug offenses. There are approximately 2 million people within the U.S. system of federal prisons, local jails, and detention centers and 75 percent do more than five years in prison.

The "War on Drugs" is costing the tax payer billions to house these convicts, and when they are released, it is difficult for them to become productive members of society, which effectively means that the average taxpayer is paying "billions" more for social services and homeless shelters for ex-convicts once they are released from prison. This is a very poor solution to the problem of drug addiction!

A benefit to getting clean and staying sober is that it significantly reduces your personal risk of becoming incarcerated.

2. Lower Risk of Injury and Disease

Many young people are not scared of death because they think "life will be over, so what do I care." Often life does not end, but major injury occurs. How many road accidents occur when people are driving drunk? If there is an accident, people can be paralyzed or sustain head injuries that do not end their life, but leave them in a compromised state for years or decades or the rest of their life.

Sadly, many addicts have poor dental health. Their teeth have decayed from smoking toxic substances and they have not been in a position to practice dental hygiene. Dentures are often required but these can be expensive so many addicts are chewing on their gums for years. This can hurt.

A person injecting heroin with a shared needle may not die of an overdose, but may get hepatitis from the needle and suffer with this disease for the rest of their life.

We had a male client in his sixties who was living homeless, drinking heavy, and using meth to keep drinking for days at a time. He had a massive heart attack that scared him straight because it did not kill him but left him feeling weaker, more vulnerable, and unable to protect himself living on the streets.

A benefit of being clean and sober is that you reduce the risk of injury and disease.

3. Lower Risk of Death

Last year, approximately 2.8 million Americans died. The cause of death to these Americans, in descending order, was heart attack and stroke 850,000, cancer 600,000, unintentional fatal injury 160,000, respiratory disease 150,000, Alzheimer's disease 120,000, drug overdose 70,000, suicide 50,000, and alcohol-induced death 35,000. Almost certainly, some deaths that are recorded as heart attack were induced by drug use and similarly with some of the 160,000 deaths by unintentional injuries were caused by drunk drivers killing innocent people whose death will have been recorded as unintentional fatal injury. Keeping the numbers simple, one out of every 30 deaths was caused by drug overdose or alcohol-induced death. One in 30, that is significant.

Overdose deaths, in descending order of most lethal drugs, were from Fentanyl, prescription opioids, heroin, cocaine, methamphetamine, and benzodiazepines. Suicide is more likely within the addict community. Clearly by removing drugs and alcohol from your life, you reduce your chances of death on many levels, directly and indirectly.

4. More Conscious and More Fun

Life is more fun without drugs and alcohol. People using drugs and alcohol may find this statement hard to believe, but this is what I have found to be true.

I love surfing, but you can substitute your preferred activities in my example of surfing. In my twenties, I would regularly smoke weed before going surfing. In my forties, I would drink beer and smoke weed before going surfing. These actions diminished my surfing abilities and make surfing far more dangerous. It is much more fun to go surfing without drugs or alcohol. I experience the event in a more conscious way and I am more present in the moment.

If you walk along the footpath above the main surf breaks in Santa Cruz, you will smell marijuana being smoked. The smell is very identifiable and strong. When I smell it, I will look around to see where it is coming from, and normally there will be a car parked 30 feet away, with some people in the car, or someone sitting on a bench, overlooking the sea, getting high. I used to be one of these people. The smell is so strong that I am very pleased that I am no longer putting that smoke straight into my lungs. It feels empowering to me to not be smoking those chemicals and to not have my brain and my mood affected by them.

Another example is playing music. I play the ukulele and I have done a few open mics. I get a little nervous before going on stage, but it feels exciting and positive. I have more control of my performance, and afterwards, I can feel the satisfaction of the experience more than if I were drinking alcohol.

By NOT using drugs or alcohol, I have more fun with each activity that I do and I do many more activities.

5. More Power and More Respect

Recently, I was in the Philippines at the birthday party of a 14-year-old boy. The boy's father is very proud of his son, so he bought a pig, which was roasted in an open pit fire for all the guests to eat. This gathering was a social success and about eight men gravitated off to one side, where there was a table and chairs in the shade away from the sun. A bottle of rum was shared around between the men. I saw this and I knew what was coming next, so I started walking away. The men called me over and said, "Come have a drink with us," and I politely said, "No thanks," and walked away. Later in the afternoon, the men were gone and I was cleaning up. There were eight empty bottles of rum! This means each man had drunk a whole bottle of rum, and if you started drinking with these men, you were expected to buy a bottle to share with the others or risk being accused of drinking without paying. The next day, I saw the father of the birthday boy. He looked sick. He was complaining about his headache and upset stomach. It took him two days to recover. There is no fun in this scenario for me.

I am very pleased to be able to avoid this type of situation and all the false emotions that go with it. I find the company of other people who are drinking to be tolerable for their first one or two drinks. They are still "normal." With more alcohol, their company becomes unbearable for me. The conversation normally degenerates into hypothetical speculations on future events and proclamations of love for anyone supporting their pontifications. With even more alcohol, the brotherly love can turn into anger toward anyone with a different opinion from theirs and intellectual exchange will melt into stupidity like butter in the hot sun.

A month after the pig-roasting birthday party, two of the men at the gathering got into a physical fight with each other because one of them believed that the other had disrespected him in some way. It seems to me that everyone at this event showed me respect for not drinking alcohol, and my experience with all the men at this gathering was positive before, during, and after the event. If you want other people to have genuine respect for you, do NOT join them in their drugs- or alcohol-consuming sessions. Set yourself apart. I am so pleased that I was able to walk away from this garbage with a polite "No thanks."

6. Consistent Thought Patterns

For me personally, there has been an increase in clarity of thought and a consistency to those thoughts that leave me feeling that I have a more meaningful life and I am more content.

216

I spend a large amount of time thinking; it has been the primary way I have made a living and it is natural for me to think about subjects from many different angles. When I was using chemicals to get high, it would cause me to "Ying and Yang" on a subject. I would go "back and forth" on a subject, "flip-flop" on a subject, and just be general undecided on subjects. Now that I am clean and sober, I have more consistent thought patterns.

A chemical high causes a high above your personal equilibrium level, and it is followed by a low below your equilibrium level, which addicts normally override by taking more chemicals. One of the biggest benefits of being clean and sober is consistently being at my natural equilibrium level.

When I go to sleep at night, I am thinking about life in a content state, and when I wake up in the morning, I am thinking about life in the same way as when I went to sleep the night before.

I am not being pulled all over the place by mood swings and shifting thought patterns. I feel that I am consistent in my thought patterns. I am "sailing with an even keel" or experiencing life in a consistent manner. This contributes to me feeling content and thankful and having a meaningful life.

7. Better Relationships

The ups and downs of chemical highs make relationships extremely difficult and impossible to keep together in the long term. Alcohol has caused more arguments, fights, and marriage breakups than any other drug. Heavy drug use brings chaos into the life of the user. Two people using have little chance of sustaining a meaningful long-term relationship. Family relationships are badly damaged by drugs and alcohol. Other people may forgive your past behavior, but don't expect them to forget about it.

It is not recommended that addicts who are new in recovery have sexual or serious relationship because the risk of relapse is too high, but having many casual relationships is important, as well as healthy, for a recovering addict. A new relationship will benefit from never having drugs or alcohol involved in the relationship. In the longer term, healthy positive relationships are going to determine the quality of your life. The more healthy positive relationships you have, the higher your personal satisfaction with life will be.

Getting clean and sober will help in the process of repairing relationships and recovery from addiction will give you more healthy, positive relationships.

8. More Meaningful Life

People ask the question, "What is the meaning of life?" The answer to this question is "Your life has the meaning that you give it."

218

If you want to get loaded all the time and die face down in a gutter, your life has had very little meaning, as measured by most standards. If you contribute to society and live surrounded by people who love you, your life has had more meaning to you and to the other people around you.

If you take a high-level view at humanity, most people are driven toward having a home and developing a family of some sort. The traditional family depicted in 1950s has been replaced by a broader definition of family, and having a home no longer means three bedrooms, two bathrooms, and a big mortgage.

Over millions of years, having a home and developing a family is the direction that the majority of humanity has taken. Getting loaded is also a common action within humanity, but it is done occasionally. The addict is the person in the group who repeatedly gets loaded to the exclusion of other healthy activities.

There is more meaning in life if the addict stops using drugs and alcohol completely and moves toward activities that give their life meaning. It is the addict who must decide the "what, how, and where" of achieving meaning in his or her life. A good starting point is to follow the lead provided by others over centuries of human existence, find a home and develop a family. If you are living at the Gault House sober home, this is your home and the people that you live with are your family.

In addition to all the benefits listed above, the recovery lifestyle involves a better standard of living, no hangovers, less feeling sick, and more money in your pocket.

Most addicts do not need a list of benefits in order to get clean and sober; they know in their heart and soul that they simply MUST overcome their addiction.

I have more respect for people who try to overcome their addiction but fail than I have for people who never try. If you try and fail, learn from your mistakes and try again. Everyone has setbacks and failures. It is important to get up and try again. It took me four or five relapses before I was successful. You have to succeed for an hour, then a day, then a month, and then six months. After six months, I felt that staying clean and sober was getting easier and I didn't have to tell myself "NO" as often, but it wasn't until I was sober for two years that I realized all the benefits of being clean and sober.

The recovery lifestyle is worth the effort; give it a try. You will have more fun and you will have a more meaningful life.

Case Study: Robert: Alcohol Old-School Style

Robert is a 61-year-old man from Southern California and a current resident of Gault House, a sober living environment. The son of alcoholic parents, he picked up his first drink at only 10 years old, malnourished and afraid and seeking an escape. His drinking led to cocaine use and jail, and finally a desire to free himself from the misery of addiction. He has been struggling toward sobriety for a long time, and has renewed his commitment to sobriety with a move to a sober living house. He currently has three months clean and sober.

Robert, how are you doing?

I'm doing great.

Why don't you tell us how you got started with your drinking.

I'm an alcoholic addict and I say that because I'm an alcoholic first and I didn't find out until much later in my life that I was an addict as well. Alcohol is my drug of choice. I have a younger sister, a year younger, and an older brother, two and a half years older. I was born in October of 1957. As I was growing up, my uncles, my aunts, and my grandparents were either Korean War veterans or World War II veterans. That's the patriarchal environment I was raised in. My dad was a hardworking guy. He moved heavy machinery in Los Angeles. He drove a truck and a trailer. The trailer was a specialized trailer and it was called a monorail.

He could pick up hundred-thousand-pound weight machines, different things, crane it onto a platform, where he can install them and disengage them. That's what he did all day long; he was a hardworking guy. He was gone whenever I got up and he would come home at 9:00 or 10:00 every night. My family looked pretty normal from the outside, looking in, I believe. Looking back, I have pictures of my brother and sister and I dressed up when we were little. I was probably four or five. I was wearing a suit. My brother was wearing a suit. My little sister is wearing a church dress. My dad had a suit on and my mom had a church dress. That was a picture that we had on the wall. I can't remember going to church too many times, but it's one of the times, I guess. Not to say we didn't, but I just don't remember too many times.

I was born in Los Angeles, California. For the first 17 years of my life, that's where I was raised. In terms of my maternal grandparents, my grandfather came over from Italy through Ellis Island in 1921. My grandmother on my dad's side came over from Scotland. She emigrated from Scotland. My paternal grandmother was a welder on the ships during World War II. She welded on the ships in San Diego and also in Brisbane, Washington. She supported herself, my dad, and his brother during the war. My dad was born in 1937. My uncle was born in 1940. My mother's family moved from Kansas City to Los Angeles, and that's where my parents met. They got married when they were 16. My dad went in the Navy immediately after getting married. He went into the Korean War when he was 16 years old. They were babies having babies.

Alcoholism and addiction is something that I'm very familiar with because I grew up with it. My dad was a drinking man beyond normal conditions. Alcoholics Anonymous or recovery programs of any kind never touched his life. He died a drinking man. I remember when he would come home from work after a long day's work. For us, bedtime was at 6:00. At 6:00, we are already bathed, fed, clean, and homework was done if we had homework. I was too young for me to have homework, but we're in bed, and my dad would come home, and I would be under the covers, waiting for him to come home. He'd come home at 9:00 to 10:00 at night. I would hear the door slam and I would jump out of bed. I would run to him and jump in his arms because that's what I wanted from my dad.

The dinner's cold and mom's pissed off and dad's drunk. He was affectionate to me for a few minutes; then he and mom started arguing, and then I became the object of his punishment. I got sent to the emergency room three times before I started kindergarten through incidents like that. Back then, the police didn't do anything about that stuff. I remember the police coming in one time and my mom pulled my pajamas down and I had bruises all over me. They looked at them and said, "Thank you, ma'am. We'll get back with you." Nothing ever happened. I talk about that because it's important later on in my story because there came a time in my life that I had to realize that nothing that happened to me mattered anymore. The only thing that mattered was that I take responsibility for my own actions, that I become accountable for my actions, and to not place the blame where it didn't belong. Life is life.

I was six years old and my brother and sister and I ended up on a plane going to Ohio. We didn't know where we were going at the time, but we ended up on a plane going to Ohio. We were going to go live with my paternal grandfather. I had only met him once in my life before this. We arrived and we had two aunts. Technically, there were my aunts, but they weren't much older than us because my grandfather had a second family. My dad, I'm going to say he was maybe 30 at the time, I could be wrong about the ages, but it's inconsequential.

My parents were getting a divorce. Nobody told us anything. We ended up on a plane and my mom didn't know where we were at. My dad took us and he put us on a plane because he wanted to hurt her. The way to hurt her the most would be to take her kids away and that's what he did unfortunately. We spent about six months there and my mom finally found out where we were. Then she came and got us.

After that, she wasn't financially or emotionally capable of taking care of us, so we lived with aunts, uncles, grandparents on both sides, different places, even strangers for a few years. When I was 10 and my sister was nine, my dad got remarried to his second wife, and he thought it was a great idea to get custody of me and my sister. I have no idea what was going through his mind about that.

He bought a house and we moved in. His alcoholism had excelled quite a bit by that time. My sister moved out after about six months, so I was there and my dad was very reactive. He was still doing the same stuff. He would beat me within an inch of my life without a moment's notice. His second wife was about as far along in her alcoholism as he was. I know this now, but I didn't know it then. I've just observed, and to the best of my memories, this is what I remember. They would come home at 5:30 every night with as much alcohol as they could carry and they'd be blacked out between 6:30 and 7:30, depending on how fast they drank.

They'd be blacked out in the living room, their heads would be tilted to the side, and I knew they were out. Sometimes there was dinner in the form of a Swanson TV dinner and sometimes there wasn't. Sometimes there was a Swanson TV dinner and they would leave it in the stove and it burned. One night when they were blacked out and there was no dinner, I went into the refrigerator. My stepmom used to keep a head of lettuce in the crisper and you could see through the glass on top of the refrigerator because there was nothing in it but beer usually, so you could see right inside the crisper. I opened up the door and I knew that if they heard me opening up the door that I would be in deep trouble.

You didn't know when the cannon was going to go off. I opened up the door real quiet. The light shined out from the refrigerator because it's dark outside about this time and there was no lettuce. I was bummed out. I was an underweight 10 year old and I was starving, but there was lots of beer in there. I reached in and I grabbed a can. It was a 16-ounce can. I remember it like it was yesterday. I was watching them the whole time. I was looking at the beer, looking at them, looking at the beer, looking at them, and listening. I took the beer to my room and shut the door. I took my shirt off and put it over the top of the beer can. It seemed like it took me 30 minutes to open the top of that beer because it was so quiet that a mouse could have heard it.

I had that thing open and I remember taking the first swig and it felt like a big guzzle of acid went down my throat. It was the carbonation. I didn't know that, but it was carbonation and probably the hops. Who knows? I waited a few minutes, the burning stopped, and I took another drink. It burned a little less. I got about half of it down and it didn't burn at all after that. I drank the rest, and I would say within 10 minutes, my stomach started getting hot and my hunger went away completely. It vanished. I had no fear. My fear went away. That alcohol took hold of me, an ounce of alcohol or whatever was in that beer can. It's an ounce and half, I guess, in 16-ounce cans. For an underweight 10 year old who was hungry, it hit me pretty fast. I went right to sleep.

That was the best thing that ever happened to me. That moment in time, in my life, I needed an escape and that was my escape. My caregivers were supposed to love and protect me. They abandoned me and hurt me. I needed relief and escape. I reflect back on that sometimes throughout my adult life and throughout my sobriety. I wonder sometimes maybe that saved my life at that very moment. There's only so much a person can take, especially a young person. I had no one to reach out to. That was it. Back then there were no cell phones. There was no easy communication to anything. At 10 years old, you don't have a support system set up for yourself. Your world is very small and it's kept small intentionally.

When I go back and I relive my life and I think about what happened and I think about where I'm at now, it gives me a lot of gratitude. If I can say anything here that helps anyone, that anybody can identify with, that helps them make that decision to live in the solution, and not live in their addiction, then this is all worth it. I get emotional when I think back on that, because it was the only relief I'd ever had in my life up to that moment in time, the present for me at that moment. Before that, I had no relief and alcohol became a solution. I didn't chase it after that and I moved out after that. I moved in with my grandparents. When I was 11, I lived with my aunt and uncle in Porterville. Then I lived with my paternal grandparents, and then with my maternal grandparents. I flipped around to just about everywhere. I ended up back with my mom a couple of times.

When I was 16, my dad was leaving a bar with his wife, and they stepped out into a crosswalk and a car hit both of them. It killed her and knocked him 40 feet, knocked the shoes right off of his feet. He was in a coma for I don't know how long. He wore a 10-inch heel on his right boot after that. That's when I was 16.

When I was 17, I went into the Marine Corps. I signed up and I went to the Marine Corps. In my family, my parents got married when they were 16. Her parents got married when they were 16. Her great-grandmother and her parents got married when they were 16. Through my family, when you were old enough to reproduce, then they figured their job was done. "You're graduating from high school. Get out of here," with no life skills, no training, no anything. That's the way they had done things. I joined the Marine Corps when I was 17 and I signed up in September of 1975.

My dad drove his pickup truck through a garage and put his face through the windshield. He had these scars about as wide as my fingers. He started below his eyebrow line and it went up all the way through his hairline right in front of his face. He walked around like that. I graduated from boot camp and came home on a 10-day leave from boot camp.

I was 17. I came home from boot camp and decided it was a great idea to get married, so me and my high school sweetheart got married, the mother of my girls. I didn't know what I was doing at the time. I thought it was a great idea because that's what my parents did and that's what everybody had done in my family. I thought that was the thing to do. Both of my parents who weren't together at the time, they were going "We'll drive you to Vegas," so they did. They drove us to Vegas. It was wonderful. But it wasn't very well thought out. My wife and I lived in Oceanside at that time. Back at that time, my first job down there was driving a truck and a trailer. I'm in the motor transport business now.

I was operating in a truck and a trailer right there on the Marine base at Camp Pendleton. I was delivering produce and food goods to all the mess halls and in tournament camps for the Vietnamese evacuees back then. I was delivering to those guys too. We got a little apartment in town. It was $125 a month back then, and it was a nice apartment. I was a PFC and I made $100 a week. That was what I got and we made it work. It was good. I got this knock on the door, about 2:00 in the morning. I opened the door. The MPs were at the door and they said, "Here, call your brother." He handed me a piece of paper that was torn off of a page. He then said, "Call your brother." They gave me his number.

I said, "What's going on?" They said, "We don't know. We were just told to come over, come and tell you to call your brother." I walked down to Thrifty's and for a dime you could make a phone call back then. I brought change. I called my brother and he said my dad had been killed. I found out that he drove his pickup truck off of Highway 2. It's called the Angeles Crest Highway. It's about a 300-foot drop. He was drinking and driving. He had 19 drunk-driving convictions at that time, two near-fatal accidents, and he was still drinking. He was still driving when he drank. Talk about a guy who didn't learn his lesson with serious trauma. To this day, the God of the universe maybe was being merciful on him to live any longer than that. He was 39 years old when that happened.

Luckily, he didn't kill anybody else after all those DUIs and stuff. You said it in the very beginning, but the state of treatment back then was so minuscule compared to the understanding we have of alcoholism and addiction today. The field didn't exist the way it does now. There wasn't much help for people.

Alcoholics Anonymous was around, but it's nothing like it is today. Addiction recovery is super-advanced these days.

My grandmother read in the newspaper that he got killed. That's the only way we knew. I had to go down to the LA County morgue and identify his body. That was something in my life that I had to accept. This program and the way that I've worked my steps, I've been able to forgive both my parents. They did the best they could. I don't give him the leeway of saying that what they did was right because it wasn't. It never would be under any circumstances. However, they did do the best with what they had and they didn't have much.

But my alcoholism progressed. When I went into the Marine Corps, my first daughter was born in May of 1978. She was about six months old and they gave me orders to go overseas. I went overseas, I went to Japan, Korea, the Philippines, and I was gone for 13 months.

As I said, there were no cell phones back then. I made two phone calls home in a year and it costs me $10 a minute on a $100-a-week salary. That's a pretty good amount of money to pay for a phone call, but it was worth every minute of it. We talked for 10 minutes each time, so it was good. That's when my alcoholism started to accelerate. I went overseas. We worked and drank. That's what we all did. Everybody who I hung out with, everybody who I knew, that's all they did. I blacked out a few times when I was over there. I got in a lot of fights.

Me and my friends, we'd like to go find other servicemen and get drunk as hell on some exotic booze. I remember the first time I drank this drink called Mojo. They call it Mojo over there in Japan. They take a fifth of every booze you can imagine, a fifth of Tequila, a fifth of vodka, a fifth of whiskey, a fifth of whatever. They all mix it up and then they put a fifth of punch in it and that's it. Then they start scooping it up and serving it to you. After a few of those, things get pretty wild.

When I came home, when I rotated back to the States, I call it the alien inside me because it changes me. I'm a Jekyll and Hyde when I drink. The alien in me, I knew it had grown. I could feel that it was something that I had to do. I'm a binge drinker. I would binge, take a break, and then binge more. Over time, my binges became closer and closer together.

After I got out of the service, I got a job out in town driving a truck and also driving a tow truck. I'm a pretty inventive guy, so I started my first business a little while after that. I started buying cars.

If I drive by a car that had dust all over it, I would pull up to the house and say, "What's wrong with your car?" They'll say, "That thing doesn't run." I'll say, "I'll buy it for $50 and tow it away right now. Give me the title." I gave him $50. It'd be a starter. I'd sell it for $1,000. Within two years, I had 25 cars parked all around my house. I'd have to move them every two days because the meter maid would come and chalk all the tires. I had a sock with about $40,000 in $100 bills in my closet. I would buy and sell cars and run my tow truck. The company I worked for had seven tow trucks. They had a nine-acre yard and they had a grandfathered auto-wrecking license that they weren't using and there was only one other in the whole county.

They had a paint booth, and they had contracts with the CHP, with the local Police Department, with the Border Patrol, all kinds of stuff going on. The two guys who owned it were old men who wanted to lose money because they had so much money they didn't know what to do with it. They needed a tax write-off, so they kept this place. I bought it off them when I was 22. That was my first business. I gave them $100,000 down and took the place over. Something clicked after that happened. I was good as long as I was buying and selling cars, but once I took that thing over, I had no idea how to run a business. I was very good at talking and getting to business, but I had no idea how to handle the administrative part of it and how to handle the different things that I didn't know. I was 22 years old, with no experience. I had no experience in life because no one taught me as I was growing up. I had no experience in business, but I knew I wanted it.

This is 1980, 1981, more or less. I don't know if you remember what happened in 1981, but tankers full of cocaine were coming over to the United States. It was almost free back then. I'd go over to anybody who I knew and they'd have a big old pile. It didn't do much for me, but it was there and I got used to it and started drinking and using it. The alcohol took away my fear and the cocaine made me feel invincible. It was a very lethal combination for me at that time in my life because I was young and full of piss and vinegar. I was 22 and I just paid $100,000 for a business. I don't know what that's worth today, but that was a boatload of money back in 1981. I got into a dispute with a couple of guys. I tried to kill one of them and they ended up sending me to prison. I got convicted of attempted murder, great bodily injury, and a gun enhancement.

I got a 14-year, four-month sentence. I ended up doing eight years and 10 months in the prison system. I went into that fast. Here I am. I'm a veteran, I own my own business, I'm young, and I'm an alcoholic and an addict. I didn't know that I was an alcoholic or an addict. I had no idea. I thought it was everybody else's fault all this time. It was always someone else, except me, because I could never be wrong. To be wrong would mean that there's something wrong with me, and I was not raised with that type of mentality.

I did my time. I have two daughters at this time. My girls were two-and-a-half and five when I went into prison and they were 10 and 13 when I got out. Their mother and I got back together when I was in the joint and we stayed together until I got out. A year after I got out I left her, and we are still dealing with that now. My oldest daughter is 42 and my youngest daughter will be 39. They were both born in May. I didn't get in any trouble before I went to prison and I haven't got into any trouble since I got out, except I got arrested for being drunk in public and I got a couple of speeding tickets, but that's about it.

It was a pretty good adjustment for me going behind bars. I didn't know anything about what it would be like to be inside. Every time I'd reflect, I'd have a couple of old cons pull me in and take me to school. They checked my heart. My heart checked good until they said, "We're going to teach you what to do here." That probably saved my life by doing that.

I went to college when I was in the joint. I was in Soledad for four years and they offered classes from Hartnell College and San Jose State University. They offered an accredited program where the professors went down to the prison and taught classes and you got credits and you graduated. I have my diploma from Hartnell College and I got my bachelor's from San Jose State. I was always doing something. The boys in the yard used to call me "Schoolboy" and I didn't care. I worked in the kitchen, so I ate as much as I wanted. I worked out every day and got healthy. That way, I was exercising my mind. I couldn't wait to get out because I wanted to be with my family. In prison, alcohol was not part of my daily life like it was on the outside.

I went to jail in February of 1982 and I got paroled in September of 1991. It's important for me to remember that alcohol is an escape for me. I needed it to turn off my head. I'm pointing toward my head here. I needed to turn off what was going on up there because it was too much for me. I couldn't handle it. Alcohol helped me do that and I turned off the pain of hunger and turned off the pain of fear. That worked at that time.

When I got out, I didn't realize that I was an alcoholic. If somebody mentioned that I had a problem with alcohol or even hinted toward that, I'd be reactive because I wasn't an alcoholic. That was saying that something was wrong with me and there's nothing wrong with me. It's got to be you. I still had that thing going on. Plus, now I've got a prison mentality, and I know it, but I can't help it because I had to live it for so long. I'm trying to get out of that deal or get away from that. I left my first wife again for the second time once I got out and remarried about seven years later, in 1997.

The woman who I married was dysfunctional. Her kids were dysfunctional. I was so blind with lust and alcohol that I couldn't see it. As a sober objective man, in the state of mind that I'm in today, I would never have made that choice, but that was then and this is now. That's where I get the gratitude from this program. The binges got closer over the years. It got closer and closer together to where I was only taking a day or two at the most after two or three weeks of pounding it down. I'd be drinking a couple quarts of vodka a day and then I would be taking Ambien. I got a prescription for Ambien. I don't know if you've ever taken Ambien, but I was taking 10-milligram pills. A 10-milligram pill will make a rhinoceros drool in about 15 minutes. I would take 10 of those a day. It was crazy.

One day, the alcohol stopped working. My body and my soul and my spirit were so poisoned. I have to explain what that means. It was obviously from the drugs and the alcohol and the abuse. Emotionally, I was bankrupt because I had never dealt with any emotional issues throughout my life. I would put the bottle to my lips and all the emotions would go away. I would never process any type of life events that happened to me. I would get pissed off, I'd drink, and I'd be over it the next day. I would forget it. I was 54 years old when all this took place. That was in March of 2012. What I didn't realize is that from the time that I was 10 and I took that can of beer until the time I was 54 years old, I hadn't dealt with much. Emotionally, I was a 10-year-old boy living in the body of a 54-year-old man. I couldn't deal with it.

Once I got introduced to this program, I realized that if I wanted to live, I needed to grow up and I needed to do it real fast. I went to this meeting of Alcoholics Anonymous at noon. A few years before that, I knew I had a problem with alcohol. I never admitted that I'd had a problem with alcohol. I even went to my doctor's a few times for a checkup. I mentioned to him maybe years before I went to my first AA meeting, I would say, "I've got a problem with drinking. Do you have a pill for that or something?" I always wanted something easy. I'd never wanted to work for it. He said, "You might want to try Alcoholics Anonymous." I'm going, "What is that? That sounds like work. Probably not. I'd rather go drink and forget it," which is what I did.

I have to say that back when I had my towing company, I had a thriving business, I turned it into a real money-maker, and then I threw it away with drugs and alcohol and then violence. Nothing changed after that, except that there wasn't violence because I knew what would happen if I did that again. I avoided violence, but I still used the escape. I started a business back in 2000. I turned it into a multimillion-dollar program and threw it away. I started another one in 2006 and I did the same thing. I started this one that I have now in August of 2010.

I went to my first meeting; it was at noon. That first meeting that I went to was important. I heard other people talk since I've been going to meetings about their first meeting. Everybody was laughing; everybody was there talking and laughing. I didn't know how I could be in a place that could help me because I felt miserable. I felt hopeless, helpless, and I didn't know what to do. These people in this room didn't sound like they had anything that I had.

Then all of a sudden everything got serious and somebody started talking. I don't remember what the speaker said. There was a speaker. I remember saying the Lord's Prayer at the end, and I started crying. I was feeling sorry for myself. I was on my pity pot feeling sorry for myself, and then I walked outside afterwards. This guy followed me out. He's from San Diego. He's not even from the area. He's from San Diego visiting. He was hitting the meeting. He followed me outside and we went to the corner. I was in the corner of the parking lot. "Do you want to smoke a cigarette?" he asked. I said, "Sure, I guess."

I didn't even smoke cigarettes. He was talking to me and said, "There's a solution. I know where you're at right now because I've been there." He started telling me a little bit about himself and he got me interested. He said, "I got the answer for you. Let's go have some coffee." We went down for two hours and read the Big Book. We were sitting right on the sidewalk in front of the coffee shop and we read the Big Book of Alcoholics Anonymous. He had me read. He wouldn't read. He said, "You need to read."

He had me read it, so it was a great exercise. After that he goes, "There's a meeting tonight right down the street at 7:00. Meet me right here on the corner and we'll go to the meeting together." I was there and he didn't think I was going to show up. To be honest with you, I didn't know if I was going to show up or not either, but I was so desperate at the time. I got the gift of desperation. I was so desperate that it was unbearable. I felt like I had bugs crawling all over my arms. When I lay down at night to go to sleep, as soon as my eyes were closed, I would start breathing like I was sleeping.

I would wake up because I was afraid I was going to stop breathing. I had that fear. There's something wrong with my middle ear. I would walk in and feel like I was walking on a rubber floor. I was pretty poisoned. My body was poisoned and my mind was poisoned. I have so many unresolved issues. I feel it when they tell the story about peeling the onion. I picture the unresolved issues that I had never dealt with through my whole life as layers of the onion. At that moment in time, I had packed so many layers into my body that no more would fit. I couldn't fit another one in there.

It wouldn't go, so I had no relief. I went to that meeting that night and these guys were coming up to me, shaking my hand saying, "My name is Jeff. What's your name?" I was thinking, "What do these guys want? This is a club and they must want to sign me up, so it's got to cost a lot of money here." This is what I'm thinking. Later on, I realized that I was so sick that anybody who knew anything could tell and see that instantly. They want to help me because it was helping themselves, but I didn't know that at the time. Jeff said, "My home group is tomorrow night." This was on a Monday.

The weekend before that, I drank so much vodka and I took so many pills that I lay on my living-room floor for 30 hours. My stepdad didn't know what to do with me. That next

Monday morning, I went to the meeting, and Jeff said, "I got my home group tomorrow night. It's in Prunedale. I'd like you to come." I said, "Okay." We exchanged numbers and I met him in Prunedale. He took me to his sponsor's house. There was a meeting at the sponsor's house. I met everybody at the meeting and I met my sponsor there.

I relapsed a whole load of times. I relapsed one day, two days, a week, six months, four months, three months. I had a million chips. Finally in March of 2012, it took. The whole thing took and I didn't drink after that. On March 2, 2012, I checked into a recovery center for 30 days. It was in San Jose. My business had 27 employees and I had 75 trucks. I signed all the checks, but I had to check out. I didn't get a phone call for 10 days and the first phone call I got was 10 minutes. I used to be connected to my phone and I had to give all that up, but I had to decide for myself what's more important,. If I wasn't sober, then nothing would exist anyways. I wouldn't have a family. I wouldn't have a business. I wouldn't have a life, and all of it would be gone and they'd be at my funeral.

When I got out of that recovery center, I had one employee left and myself. I started to rebuild my company. I told my creditors the truth. I owed the federal government $350,000. I hired a tax attorney who got me an offer and a compromise. Many good things happened after that. It was unbelievable. Because I was telling the truth, some of the customers I called before I went into that recovery thing said, "Go ahead and take care of yourself." They already knew it. They already know I had a problem. When I got out, when I would talk to other people, I found out that there are other people who are recovered too in my business. I met a new guy. I've known this guy for 25 years. He's got two years of sobriety right now. Back in the heyday, he was horrible like me. We both talk about it all the time and we do business together. We know what we get when we deal with each other. We get the good stuff.

I accepted the difference between all those times that I tried to get sober, even though I wanted to. Even though I was desperate and even though I did the steps and I did all the work that I was asked to do, I didn't have a higher power that I relied on. I hadn't admitted to my innermost self that I was an alcoholic and that my life was unmanageable. I knew my life was unmanageable, but I didn't admit to my innermost self that I was an alcoholic addict. The moment I did that and the moment I started relying on a higher power on a daily basis, it was easy. I didn't have a drink after that. I got in with the program. I had to reprogram the entire way I lived my life into a different way of living.

There were no more lies, no more dishonesty. Everything was being sanitized with the sunlight of the spirit. When people came to me and said, "You did this and you did that," I wasn't backpedaling saying, "If I admit this, then I'm admitting that I'm doing something wrong and I'm never wrong." All that crap had to go out the window. I'm saying, "I remember that, and that was wrong for me to do that. I don't do that anymore. How can I make that right? Do I owe you money? Do I owe you labor? Let's make that right."

This disease is an allergy of the body and an obsession

of the mind. I could not stop thinking about escaping my life. I equated that with drinking alcohol because that's exactly the first thing that happened when I took my first drink. It was an escape from reality through alcohol. It was instantaneous. About nine months into the program, I was talking to a friend who got sober almost at the same time as me, about six days after me. We were talking outside of a meeting and then I'm going, "I don't remember the last time I wanted to drink off of my problems. I don't know when that happened, but I know it's gone. It's a miracle." I lived my entire life like that, and all of a sudden, I was free from it. It was such a wonderful gift.

I wanted to tell everybody. It was like the church guy who gets Jesus and he runs around the pews because he's so excited about it. That was me at Alcoholics Anonymous. I jumped on that pink cloud and I stayed on it. I stayed on it. I stayed sober.

Some other funny things happened. I started taking care of my body. I was 255 pounds. I started exercising, taking vitamins, eating the right food, and doing the right things. My stepdad had a quadruple bypass surgery and I was able to take care of him during that and able to be there and be present for him. It was great because he's been in my life since I was 14. After I was sober for four-and-a-half years, I thought I should check my cholesterol. I should start checking this stuff. I went and had an MRI on all my arteries. They came back with a disc. The disc said, "0 percent of the population has less plaque than you in your arteries." I couldn't believe that. I had been taking fish oil and krill oil and exercising every day for four-and-a-half years. Who knows what I looked like inside before that, but this is what I look like now.

A few months later, I was wearing these glasses and my vision was getting worse. I was going, "t's time to go get some new glasses. Something's going on here." I go into my optometrist. I've had the same guy for 10 years or longer than that, maybe 20 years now. I go into the optometrist, he puts me in the thing, puts the drops in, looks in my eyes, scopes it out. He goes, "What have you been doing?" I weigh 195 at this time. I lost 60 pounds and I kept it off. I'm going, "I'm taking my vitamins and eating good food and exercise on a regular basis." He goes, "Whatever you're doing is right. Your right eye used to be your bad eye." I had better-than-average vision in my left eye and I barely had any in my right eye. He said, "You need reading glasses; that's all you need." My vision improved. Who gets that when they're my age?

My cardiovascular health improved; everything improved. My life got better; my kids got back into my life. It was a wonderful thing. I was able to help people. I did everything I was supposed to do and life was wonderful. I have two service commitments. I went to the psych ward at the local hospital for four years. I went to Soledad Prison, where I did time, and saw a couple of guys who I knew. These are guys who are doing life and will never get out. They know what we know. It was funny. That was unbelievable that I saw that. I thought about that before I took that commitment and I said, "I was in for a while. There's got to be somebody in there who's still in there who wasn't there when I was there." It gave me gratitude.

Those guys in there are like we are. There's no difference in their addiction than what we have. They get it. The guys who go to those meetings, they want help. I felt grateful that I could take the message to them and then present it as someone who knows where they're at because I was there. I have several service commitments. I have a home group. I had a group of men who I kept in contact with. I did everything I was supposed to do. Whenever I had fear, I could call somebody and I could talk to someone. One of the guys who I knew more likely had already gone through what I was about to go through. The miracle of the whole program is that I didn't have to do this alone.

There were other people who have been through what I had been through. They already had been through what I'm going to go through in the future. They could help with that. I didn't have to escape or run from anything. If I had a medical issue, I'd see a doctor. If I had a legal issue, I went to an attorney. If I had a tax issue, I'd go to a tax lawyer. If I had a spiritual issue, I would go to AA. I would talk to my sponsor. Being able to do an inventory on different things, no matter what it is, you can break it down and see what part belongs to me and what part doesn't and be willing to accept that.

Have you kept the same sponsor over your entire time in recovery?

No. I've had three sponsors. The original sponsor who I had, I had him up until I went into that recovery center. When

I came out of that, I got another sponsor. I was sober about six-and-a-half years. I got sober on March 2 of 2012 and then I took a drink around October of 2018. Whatever that is, it was quite a bit of time and most of it I enjoyed. January or February of 2018, I made a decision in my professional life and it was a wrong decision. I made it for the wrong reasons and I was unwilling to take it back. My pride and my ego got in the way. In order to fix it, I started pouring myself in my business. I made a choice when I did that to put my business before my sobriety. That was another thing that I did when I took my last drink. I made my sobriety the absolute most important thing in my life, and then all that changed. It was fear-based. I lost a whole lot of money and instead of being humble and admitting my faults, I decided not to do that.

I got resentment from another member of this program. Then I got resentment from a family member and then from a business associate. I didn't resolve any of them and they ground me up inside. If I had come clean with the whole thing and gave it back and said, "I was wrong. Let's start over," but I can't go back. It happened. I ended up taking a drink in October of 2018. It took me about 10 months to take that drink from the time that I made that decision. A whole series of events took place and I'm going to tell you the disease is alive and well in me. It's waiting patiently and it knows my weakest moment. That's when it's going to grab onto me and it won't let go. It says, "Hate on him. Hate on her. You don't need to go to that meeting today," and all of a sudden, a drink doesn't seem so bad until you take it and then it runs away with your understanding, your soul, your life.

June 27 was my last drink. I got so many days in my new recovery program and I feel like the years that I was sober did not go to waste whatsoever. I have all those tools in my toolbox now. It felt like I went to sleep for a while and I woke up again realizing what's important in my life. Without this program, the fellowship, and my higher power, I won't have anything else. Everything else will disappear as it has for so many, as it did for my dad. I believe he felt hopeless and helpless. "People don't know what the solution is. They end up driving off a cliff." I had no idea that my dad did drive off a cliff when he said that. I relate to stuff these days. Instead of picking out the differences, I find the similarities and that's what keeps me connected to everything.

What advice would you give to someone who's maybe considering getting sober or has been sober and has gone back to drinking again?

For the newcomer, for those who know deep down inside that you have a problem with alcohol or drugs of any kind, in chapter three of the Big Book of Alcoholics Anonymous, it says that our disease always gets worse and it never gets better. That's absolutely true for everyone who I know. I know thousands of people in this program who I've met throughout the years. Every one of them says the same thing—it always gets worse and it never gets better. That statement is true. It's true and is tested in time.

You don't have to live that way. You don't ever have to take a drink or a drug again in your whole life. Even if you want to take it, you don't have to take it. Those of you who are unsure, there are a lot of ways to test it. There's a 20-question pink questionnaire that Alcoholics Anonymous gives out. You don't need to show it to anybody. You can answer them in private yourself, but be honest when you're answering it. If you check enough of those boxes, maybe you need to look into it. The other thing is go to a bar and take one drink. That's it. Leave and then not take another alcoholic drink for another month. Maybe you're not an alcoholic and you can do this, but if you find that you cannot complete this test for whatever reason, maybe you are an alcoholic.

I know what this program has done for me, and I know where I was at when I got here. I wasn't looking for a club to join, to upgrade my professional life or my pleasure life. I was desperate. I was seeking a solution. I was desperate to seek the answer that I was looking for and I didn't know what it was. I wanted to quit drinking, but I didn't know how. I had a reason to get drunk my entire life. I always made up a reason, and at the end, I didn't have any reason. It's just what I did. I got drunk. With drinking comes lies, deception, everything that destroys, all the destructive mechanisms that go with it.

I've heard throughout the years people talk about the seven-year itch and the five-year itch and all this stuff. I would say that I got too comfortable with who I was. I had no desire to drink. I could go anywhere where everybody could be drunk and I wouldn't want it. It wouldn't cross my mind, but I got too comfortable. I was protected because my higher powers protected me because I was doing what I was supposed to do. I was pouring that protection over me on a daily basis. I was saying my prayers every morning. I was asking to be under his protection and care, directing my thoughts and my actions on a daily basis. I was giving myself up to him in the third-step prayer on a daily basis so I could be an example for others or for whoever cared to look.

I stopped doing that. I made something else my priority. I needed this evidently. On the June 28, I ended up in the emergency room and it took me nine days to get there. I was drinking. The whole thing about it was that my body was clean and I was 60 pounds lighter than when I stopped drinking, but in my brain, my mind told me that I could drink as I did before. I was consuming as much alcohol as a 255-pound man could drink, but I was a 195-pound man and it put me on my ass. These friends of mine who were in the apartment complex next to me, they were downstairs. He and his wife came into the ER, into the room, because they heard that I was over there and they walked in the room and they didn't recognize me. They said, "We didn't even recognize you." I suggest anybody who wants to be free of the obsession and the allergy, there is a solution.

Robert, thank you so much for sharing your story.

Chapter 12: Additional Case Studies

Below are several additional case studies that I hope will reinforce the message that addiction affects many people and it is a serious problem to which we should give serious attention. Some names have been altered to protect the privacy of those individuals. These case studies are interviews with addicts who have lived at Gault House.

1. Elijah: Male, 26, Alcohol and Cocaine, dead at 27-years-old
2. Clara: Female, 23, Alcohol, Cocaine, Heroin with boyfriend
3. Ivy: Female, 43, Alcohol and Pills in Hawaii and Lake Tahoe
4. JJ: Male: 42, Alcohol and Everything Else
5. Kendra: Female, 34, Homeless on Heroin
6. Michelle: Female, 29, Alcohol while working at Nordstrom
7. Andrea: Female, 43, Mother on Meth
8. Billy: Male, 55, Meth leads to Gangs & Prison
9. Heather: Female, 28, Cocaine at the District Attorney's Office
10. Amanda, Female, 26, Alcohol and Cocaine, Spiral of Addiction

If you prefer to listen to these case studies, an audio version of them is available on the Podcast page of our website:

www . ResponsibleRecovery . net

1. Elijah: Male, 26, Dead at 27 Years old

Elijah is a 26-year-old Oregonian who began smoking pot as a sophomore in high school. He soon began drinking and eventually turned to cocaine, which took over his life. Unable to hold on to a job and grappling with mental health concerns, he is newly sober (13 days at the time of recording) and a resident at Gault Street Sober Living Environment. He has never been to a treatment facility and is determined to hold on to his mental clarity through sober living.

Eli, how are you doing?

I'm good. Thank you.

Please tell us how your addiction got started?

I didn't start using until right around the beginning of my sophomore year in high school. I've always been interested. I always hung out with the other kids who smoked a lot of weed and drank too. It was only something that I was intrigued by. I didn't necessarily have the motivation to do it. I didn't feel compelled to do it until I hit an episode of depression. I was going through a very bad existential crisis. There's a back story behind that too that I don't mind talking about either. It was a pretty bad one.

What happened?

I used to be part of this youth group at this church here in Santa Cruz on Mission Street. It's called the Christian Life Center. We had a wonderful man. His name was Pastor Kyle. He led the youth group. He did a great job of teaching us the scripture in a way we could understand. It wasn't done in a very intimidating way. Especially the older people, the older generation, they've had some intimidating, almost authoritative, figures who were heads of the church. They had a guilt-based sermon, but he did not. His was based on the possibilities of greatness through faith. He was given a job offer up in Washington State as the head pastor. It has better pay. It's appropriate for him because he was trying to raise a family. I don't think that he considered Santa Cruz to be a very good family town.

He immediately took the job. That was something that was hard for me to deal with because I looked at him as such a great guy, almost a father figure in some ways. I felt that it was the best way to cope with the depression that followed. It was a combination of depression and an existential crisis because a lot of my faith was reinforced by him and his presence and his teachings. That was something I wasn't very good at dealing with losing that. I've had a lot of instances in my life where I've been let down by father figures or males. It was a very tough thing to deal with.

Right at the beginning of that period of depression and existential crisis, I said, "Screw it." I remember the first night pretty vividly. My friend and I went up to his house and we smoked. It was a pretty awful night because what happened was we ended up walking into somebody else's house. We had eggs thrown at us. I was wearing this jacket that my grandparents got me. It said, "Propaganda" on the back and it had backward letters. I don't know if you know what Cyrillic is, but it's basically Russian spelling. Some of the letters are backwards. I was very disappointed because that was a very cool jacket that I've had.

I didn't immediately want to drink. What happened was I realized that marijuana was making me paranoid. I was like "How am I going to combat that? I'll drink some alcohol." I remember my first drink was champagne and this was a couple of days before New Year's Day. I don't remember exactly what day it was, but it was sometime in the month of December of that same year. It was November when I first used, and then in December, I ended up drinking for the first time.

What happened after that?

The same thing pretty much happened. I grew fond of smoking and drinking. It got to the point where I needed it. I needed it in order to feel happy. Keep in mind that in the midst of all this, I was dealing with my existential crisis. It was a way to suppress those fears of not knowing what happens, not knowing why we're here. It can drive people crazy. I felt that it was the best way to suppress it. It did help, but as I've come to learn, to this day, it's putting a Band-Aid on it, a wet Band-Aid, because it's not going work.

Your friends, did they use the same amount or the same stuff you did? Where were you at in terms of your friends' group and how much do you guys all use?

I would say that we're probably on the same level. It took me a while to get to their level for sure. I was somebody who was timid at first, but then it got to the point where I was like " was smoking more than them." Even they were like "You've got to take it easy." There was an incident where we had shoulder-tapped and we got a bottle of Jack Daniels, one of those big ones. I don't know how much it is. We ended up taking it back to my friend's house with another friend. We drank and we smoked. I remember waking up in the morning and having the big toenail off of my right big toe missing. There was a pretty nasty scar. There was a wound there. They said, "Last night you felt motivated to kick the cement curb. You had flip-flops on." Immediately, I was like "Oh, God." Then I went to the toilet and picked my cuts out.

Were you blacked out when you kicked the curb?

Yes, I still don't have any recollection of it. I don't think I am. That was many years ago.

An interesting thing I've seen, it's like a hallmark of alcoholism or at least the potential to develop alcoholism, is if you have a propensity to black out when you drink. Did that happen frequently when you would drink or drink excessively?

It didn't happen every time, but it certainly happened occasionally. It took me a while to black out after that because I got sent away to a boarding school. After I graduated, I'd say about eight or nine months, I was at my house with my mom and my stepdad. We all lived there. I was drinking some vodka. I literally passed out onto my back and I apparently threw up. I was lucky enough for my mom to hear me and she ended up flipping me over on my side, pretty much saving me there.

You said you got sent to a boarding school. What happened around that?

There was a lot leading up to this, because in my sophomore year, I changed high schools. I initially went to Soquel High School. I had legitimate problems there. I was dealing with somebody who was a bully and a stalker. I didn't do anything to make the situation better, because I got a little kick out of it, like a cat-and-mouse game. I didn't take it as seriously as my folks did. My folks said, "We don't feel comfortable when you're going to school. We're going to move you to Santa Cruz High." Santa Cruz High was much worse in terms of the crowds. It was very polarized. There were either straight-A students or people who love ditching class, smoking, drinking, and stuff. I'm sure there's much more going on, but that was where I was at my level there. Toward the end of that year, that was sophomore year, I played hooky. I was a truant. When I came back to Santa Cruz High at the beginning of junior year, I was basically a truant in every other class. I don't know what happened behind the scenes. I'm sure they threatened expulsion with me. They ended up saying, "We've got to do something." They sent me away.

What was a boarding school like?

It was very rewarding. It certainly taught me a lot about dealing with people. It was very difficult to develop very good social skills when I was smoking and drinking. Even before then, I was completely sober through middle school and elementary school, but I was never a very social kid. I was always very socially awkward and socially anxious. It wasn't something that I had ever learned until at that point in my life, which is late for some people. I'm grateful that I at least had the opportunity. A lot of things happened at the boarding school, where I got a whole new perspective on things. I realized that you can't always get what you want. It's a cliché, but it's true. You've got to learn how to accept defeat sometimes.

It's definitely a lesson in that. Was it a behavior role reason you went there or was it because of the crowd you're hanging out with or is it because you weren't going to class periodically?

It's a combination of reasons. It was the alcoholism. It was marijuana. It wasn't necessarily marijuana abuse. What I thought was more of my problem at that stage was the alcohol. Marijuana came second, but I'm not trying to promote marijuana with the problems people have with that. In that instance, my family was especially concerned because we've had alcoholism in our family. Two of my uncles or great-uncles specifically have died of alcohol-related diseases. They always said, "You shouldn't drink because of what happened to your Uncle Ron and your Uncle Bobby." It was a combination of reasons. It was also the fact that I wasn't very social. I didn't know how to interact with people. But definitely behavioral, the way I interacted with my family. I was in a position where I was an only child and I was spoiled beyond what I actually deserved. They even said that regrettably, "I think we spoiled him a little too much." That was one thing I had to learn. You've got to work for certain things. You've got to put in the work for sure.

It sounds like you had a good experience there and learned a lot. What happened when you came back to Santa Cruz?

I didn't take much out of it at first. I was so grateful to be home and able to smoke weed and drink again. It wasn't until years later that I started applying some of those skills and some of those lessons I learned in boarding school. I wasted a lot of time there. Things were going good at boarding school, but things didn't start to take off until five years later in 2015. I was unemployed for the most part. My family was still enabling me. They knew what was going on. I was smoking a lot of weed, drinking a lot, playing a lot of video games, and I wasn't doing anything with my life. I don't regret it either because I feel I've got it all out of my system at this point. It's unfortunate that it had to be that way, but it is what it is honestly.

I've been in a similar position myself and seen it in a lot of people. I figure, at least in your early twenties and certainly in the teenage years, if you're going to put off getting to work, better you do it when you're in your thirties or forties. You've got more to lose basically in it. Although if your family is enabling you, if they're helping put a roof over your head, then at least you're not sleeping outside or something.

That was something I am always grateful for. That's the reason why I don't feel deep feelings of regret. Of course, it's better late than never. I feel that if anything, it has given me a testimony to other people, to other kids. If I could send a message out to the youth now, I would say, "Don't waste any time. Don't sit on your hands because there are a lot of things to do. Trust me—it's a lot more fun to be working than it is sitting at home." It seems like it's fun, but it's a false sense of fun. You're not achieving anything. It's best to go out, get a job, have a social life, and see where that takes you.

When you're making money too, there's a sense of accomplishment at the end of the day when you've been working that is really rewarding. Where did the cocaine come into play?

I did my first line of cocaine in late 2015. This is coincidentally after I got my first real job. I was working at a grocery store in Santa Cruz, a health food store. I had reconnected with an old childhood friend of mine who was a big smoker and drinker all the way back to middle school. We knew he did it, but I never partook with him. I was with another group of friends at that point, but we had reunited. He was the one who introduced me not only to cocaine, but also methamphetamine and MDMA. He certainly wasn't a good influence on me. It was hard because we were good friends and having that time apart and then reconnecting, we were like making up for lost time. It's like "We never did this before. I would always be high and you would always not be high. Now we're both high." It's faulty logic, but we didn't care. It was a friendship thing; it was a bonding thing.

What did your use look like?

I couldn't quantify it back then because he was the one buying it. I'd give him money and he would go buy some. It wasn't until 2016 that I started buying it myself. I started out by doing grams. I'd go through those very slowly because I do very tiny lines as most users do. They start out small. A year later, I started bumping it up. I would do eight balls and that would usually last me a week and then going further even a year, it would be an eight ball at night.

Would you combine that with drinking?

Absolutely—It was a vicious cycle. What would happen is I would go to the bars and start drinking. Then after I got a buzz or even got drunk, then I thought do you know what sounds good? If I had some cocaine right now, I'd get that. I'd end up doing a lot of cocaine. If I had worked the next day, I would say, "I've got to get to sleep." I would drink to put myself to sleep and it worked. It's a trap that people fall into. It's like "I'm still working. I'm functioning." I'd wake up in the morning because I would be hungover. I'd do some coke, go to work, and then the whole thing would start right over.

Did people know? Did you ever get comments from people about how you look the next day?

I think so. I think that they noticed, but they never said anything. I think they were afraid to address the subject with me because admittedly I was an erratic person when I was strung out. That's not something that they wanted to have to deal with, especially in the workplace because we're all there to work. We're not there to work out our personal stuff. What made it difficult was the fact that most of my coworkers did cocaine. We were in the restaurant industry together and we would work pretty long hours. We would be scheduled and in blocks of eight hours, but it would always end up being very busy at random times. We'd say, "I got a 12-hour shift, and I've got to do a bump to keep me going."

That's what made it difficult. Many people in my workplace were doing it. That certainly made me feel better about my use. I was like "That's probably part of the reason why they're not addressing it." In my mind, I was like "Everything's cool. I'm fine." Then it got to the point where I wasn't even going to work. I was calling in sick and sometimes I wouldn't call. It would be a no call, no show. That's eventually what led to my firing, which I feel is where I started to hit my very low point.

What happened at that point when you got fired?

I had turned 25 right before I got fired. I was able to access a custodial account that was put in my name. It was a trust that had a lot of money in it. That's when my addiction got out of control. That's when I started doing the eight-ball night because I felt like "I've got all this money." That lasted for a good long year, maybe even a year and three months. That was probably my low point for an entire year, in 2018, and I didn't do anything. I didn't work at all. I did nothing but do drugs and drink a lot. It was pretty sad. I didn't feel happy doing it, to be honest. Honestly, I did it because I didn't know what else to do. I didn't think that I had any other purpose in life. I told myself, "I don't care if I die doing this. I got nothing else anymore." It was a rough time.

Were you still living with your folks at that point?

No. Two months after I got fired, we had to move out because the owner of the house we were renting wanted to retire. I don't know what she did with the house. One of her family members was living there, but we had to go because she didn't want to do the property manager duties anymore. That's when I moved back into a place that I had lived at on and off since 2012. The thing that was very difficult about that was the fact that people at that house were people who liked to do what I did. They pretty much turned a blind eye, which didn't discourage me from doing anything. It actually encouraged me to do more.

Did your parents know how bad your drug use was getting toward the end?

Yes, they definitely knew. What would happen is I would have all my bags on my floor. My room was an absolute pigsty. What would happen is I'd walk around barefoot and a bag would catch on the bottom of my foot. I'd go out into the common area like the kitchen or the living room, and they would find all these bags all over the place. I was so strung out that I didn't care. I think they knew they couldn't change my mind. I was going to do what I was going to do. It was pretty hard for them to deal with it.

What happened at the very end? What led you to wanting to change?

I have been working at this job for about several months in a couple of days. Things have been going well, but keep in mind, my addiction carried on into that job. I got clean for a while and then I started using it again. I did it with so much caution that I never ever used before I went into work. It is the same with drinking or smoking. I never did any of that. This would always be at night. It wasn't like any amounts that I was doing before. Even if I did do that eight ball in the night, it would be on my weekends, so it wouldn't affect my work. Then I thought, I don't think that this is going to take me anywhere. At first, when I started using cocaine, I was into it. I enjoyed it, but it got to the point where I was doing it to feel normal. That's what I've learned. I shouldn't ever want to do anything or put anything in my body that's going to make me feel different.

I've heard often and you also said that the restaurant industry is rife with drug and alcohol abuse. They used stimulants to keep going and work long shifts, then drink to come back down. It matches exactly your story. I wonder, how has it been for you working in that area while not using it?

It's been a lot better because I've found different ways to keep going. The workplace that I'm in now, the people are much more pleasant than the previous place where I got fired. That definitely helps when you're dealing with people you don't like, but if you're coked-out, you can tolerate them a little more. At least that's the way I used it. I used it to calm me down in some ways, but at the same time, calm me down with people who I didn't like, but also to stimulate my body to keep going. It's a weird thing, but that's the way I used it. The current workplace where I'm at, I get along with everybody. They like me over there, and I feel I have too much to lose to continue using. Even if it's a small amount, even if it's a little bit on my weekends, I don't want to take any chances because I know what happened at my previous job when I did that. That's how it started. I was like "I'm doing a little bit on the weekends. I'm doing a little bit right before I go to bed. It's not going to affect my work." I don't know. I don't necessarily trust myself with that type of thing anymore.

It sounds like you have the support of your coworkers. I think that can be helpful. You don't want to let people down. It ties in with that sense of accomplishment when you know you've done a good job after working for a day. What are your hopes for the future? You're one of our newest residents here at Gault House. You've certainly done really well since you moved in. I'm wondering what your outlook looks like, how you hope to turn your new-found recovery into something more.

Especially the younger crowd, I want to let them know that drugs and alcohol are not the answer. In terms of making yourself feel good or feeling competent, you need to have things in your life like a job, a skill, a hobby, or a relationship with the family. It doesn't matter. Basically, anything that gives you confidence. The best high, in my opinion, is being high on life. Not having to rely on material things, like drugs and other things too. I'm sure there are other bad vices out there as well.

How about sex and gambling?

I never got into either of those. There's so much more to life than drugs. With drugs and alcohol, they limit your ability to experience life to the full effect. You can't experience it the full way that you can when you're sober. I didn't use my first substance until my sophomore year of high school. Sobriety is not necessarily too much of a foreign thing for me. I did have some good times back before I started using, even if I had a lot of anxiety and a lot of depression. But I did have some good times, and that's something that I'm starting to experience again. It's the joys of human interactions. Customer Service is something that I like. I love seeing happy customers. That makes me feel so good. I would say it's letting other people know that you don't have to be trapped in addiction, that you can get out of it. It's important that you do not do it just for yourself, but if you've got loved ones around you, especially if you've got a family that has invested a lot in you, and you don't want to let them down. If you have kids, you can't raise a family if you're using drugs. Even if you are, they're going to end up in a very bad place.

I would also say it seems difficult at first. It's a daunting task to stop using, but continuing using is even more difficult and hard on us. But you can't see that when you're trapped in the midst of addiction.

I'm glad you're here, Eli. You're able to stop using and I appreciate you doing this. Thank you, Eli, for joining us and sharing your story of addiction. And to our readers, we wish you to stay sober and to be happy.
<u>**Update:**</u>

Elijah had been sober for almost three weeks at the time of this interview, which was done on Tuesday, October 8, 2019. Elijah moved out of Gault House on January 15, 2020, and the management team recorded this note for his reason for departure; "He decided to move out of his own accord; he didn't seem to take the program seriously."

Unfortunately, the Santa Cruz Sentinel Obituaries stated on Friday, March 20, 2020, that "Elijah Robert Perez Palma died suddenly and unexpectedly; he was 27 years old. We believe that his cause of death was related."

2. Clara, Female, 23 Alcohol, Cocaine & Heroin, Boyfriend's Money

Clara is 23 years old and she is currently a student. Clara found Gault House in Santa Cruz through Craigslist and this is her second stay there.

Welcome Clara, how did your addiction start?

My addiction started when I was around 16 and I started smoking pot. I always thought It's just weed. Everybody told me, "It's a gateway drug," and I pretty much thought that was bullshit. I basically started smoking because I was always really insecure growing up. I have Turrets and it was really bad when I was young. I didn't so much yell things as like make small noises. I had a lot of weird twitches and compulsive behaviors. I was very insecure about that growing up because kids pointed it out. When I finally found an outlet through smoking weed, I felt edgy and I found friends through that. Even if you have nothing else in common, if you do the same drug, there you go. That's pretty much where I started.

I started drinking when I was maybe about 16 or 17. It was around the same time. I always had this obsessive feeling to push myself as far as I could possibly go. I would drink until I passed out and then I'd wake up and just want to drink some more. I didn't think it was a problem until I was about 20.

I went through a bad breakup when I was 19. I cheated on this amazing guy with a mutual friend of ours. The whole situation was fucked up, and I felt so guilty and so shameful about it that I decided I needed to punish myself. That was when I started drinking alcoholically.

I wasn't 21 yet, so I'd get somebody I worked with to buy me a bottle of Jameson or vodka or something and then I would just drink until I passed out. Or I'd go out to a party and drink until I blacked out and end up naked and confused somewhere. I definitely think that my addiction started when I was about 16, but it didn't escalate until I was about 19 or 20.

Why do you think you used drugs?

To fit in was a huge part—at least that's where it started. After a while, it became a punishment. After it stopped being a punishment and I realized that I couldn't stop, it was to drown out the feelings I had. I hadn't made amends to anybody. I had done so many shitty things to people when I was fucked up. It became a way to escape all the shame I felt and a way to keep hating other people because if I was always fucked up, so I never had to go and deal with things. I didn't have to deal with the fact that I slept with my friend's boyfriend and ruined their relationship or all the horrible things I've said to people, just screamed in their faces over petty small things that weren't a big deal. I had so much anger I wanted to get out. I was so angry at myself and I hated myself so much that it spilled over onto other people.

What drugs did you use and how often did you use them?

My drug of choice is alcohol. I generally use it every night until I am too hungover to keep using. With alcohol, it was usually a cycle of drink until I pass out, wake up, keep drinking, if I could, or wake up, and be so viciously hungover that I was in bed for two days, throwing up until I was weak. I felt like a shriveled shell of a person. It was horrible. After a while, I started doing cocaine because honestly that way I could drink more. That escalated very quickly. I was unemployed at the time, so I was doing it most every night up until the morning. If I wasn't too hungover and sick, I would buy the next day.

I was dating this guy, and whenever he bought it, I would pretty much do all of his too. If it was in front of me, I was going to be doing as much as I possibly could. After a while, I went to my first rehab. It was really helpful. I stayed sober for about two months and then I started dating somebody else. He overdosed on heroin. We still stayed together after that. After a while, I relapsed on alcohol. We both were kicked out of our sober living environments. That was when I did heroin for the first time and I was really drunk when I did it. He took the needle off of a syringe and he shot it up my nose and I remember begging him to shoot me up. He refused because I was hammered and he kept telling me, "You'll die if I do that." I told him, "Who cares? It's fine. I'm not going to die, and if I do, whatever. I'm fucked up. It doesn't matter to me if I die because I'll be dead. Fuck my family and all the people who love and care about me." I wanted to die. I didn't care about living. At least I didn't when I was in that state of mind.

I did heroin maybe four or five times. It's honestly hard to keep track. I never shot it up. He always pumped it up my nose. Every single time, I begged him to shoot me up. After that, we went to his parents' cabin. I got really drunk, and the next morning, we were supposed to meet up with his parents, but instead, I decided that I would steal their bottle of vodka and drink until I blacked out again. We left and did not meet up with his parents. We drove back to Santa Cruz, and this is when I started to break down after this run. I woke up and we were somewhere in Santa Cruz. I didn't know where we were, but I knew exactly why we were stopped there. I turned to him and I said, "What are you doing? Why are we here?" He said, "I'm buying drugs." I remember screaming at him, calling him like a worthless drug addict. I punched him in the face and it was unbelievable that I could say these things while being drunk, after everything that I had already done. Eventually, I calmed down, and after I calmed down, I said, "Go buy drugs because I want to do them."

How did you afford your drugs? What did you do to get your drugs?

I spent all my savings on cocaine. That was pretty much how I did it at the time. After that, I had to slow down. That's why I always went back to alcohol because it's cheap and I can always afford alcohol. I could always get together enough money or change. My dad has this huge bowl of quarters in his office and I would take all of his quarters and go buy alcohol. As far as the cocaine went, I spent all my money on it, ended up getting another job, and spend everything I made at that job on cocaine. I stole from my parents and I felt so guilty about that.

When I was doing heroin, my parents had given me a little bit of money. They were supporting me at the time because I was supposed to be in recovery. I spent all the money they had given me on alcohol and drugs. The guy I was dating also spent all the money his parents had given him. It's like we were these spoiled loved children who took what their parents had given them and proceeded to destroy their lives. It was really, really unfair to my family. I would work as much as I could. I still called in sick often because I was hungover so often. I worked as much as I could and I spent pretty much every last dime on getting fucked up.

What caused you to turn around your drug use?

I was tired of wanting to die. I thought a lot about killing myself for a while. I had a lot of prescription drugs and there were multiple times when I looked up how many pills is it going to take to kill me. There was a night where I half-assed tried to hang myself. I wanted to die, but I just couldn't do it. I was tired of that. I was tired of feeling like a piece of shit all the time. I was tired of not living up to the potential that I know that I have. I'm a smart person. I'm a hard worker. I'm kind and I'm good to people, but only when I'm sober. I knew that while I was fucked up. Just knowing that, that I had that potential, that's what drove me to go to the three rehabs that I went to, The Camp, Janus, and Santa Cruz Residential (SCR).

What did your early recovery days look like?

I'm in early recovery now. I've got a few days. I'm anxious, afraid, and I have a lot of those obsessive-compulsive tendencies that are coming back because I can't drown them out. I'm focused and I'm not flaking on people. I'm able to see a future for myself.

What do you believe are the keys to recovering from addiction?

I think honesty, being honest with yourself, being honest with others, owning up to the things you did wrong. It takes a lot of courage to recover. That courage can falter and that's when you relapse. Relapse is definitely a part of my story, but it's having the courage to keep coming back, even though it didn't work before, not giving up.

What's your opinion of the 12-Step Program?

The 12-Steps are awesome, honestly. People don't understand them. I definitely didn't before I was in the program. I thought it was a cult. I was raised very religiously and I had a lot of resentments against God and anything concerning God. Coming into the program and really seeing the kinds of people who worked the 12-Steps and the way that you can work them and do them right, but also be true to yourself, it's a "God of your own understanding." In my opinion, you can be an atheist and work the 12 Steps.

What worked for you in recovery?

For me, the tenth step is very important; doing a daily inventory. I'm looking at the things that I did or thought or felt that day that could possibly be a risk. It's important to catch things early. I isolate. When I start to catch myself isolating, I try to nip it in the bud. Self-awareness is extremely important because it's you—you're in control of your program. Nobody's going to force you to be sober. You can get a sponsor and they'll support you, but that's all they can do. It's you—you have to be accountable.

Tell me what your future looks like?

I'm looking forward to starting school. I had wanted to go to school for years and years and I've dropped out four times because I had other things to do. I'm looking forward to expanding my knowledge, challenging myself, challenging my intelligence. There are so many things that I'm interested in and so many things that I could be capable of now that I'm sober, now that I'm present. Who knows, political science or archeology or literature. These are things I love and care about but I never had time for before. I'm excited about it.

Clara, thank you so much for joining us and sharing your story of addiction. And to our readers, we wish you to stay sober and happy.

3. Ivy: Female, 43, Alcohol, Pills & Relationships, Hawaii and Lake Tahoe:

Ivy is 39 years old and works at a health spa. Ivy was born and raised in Hawaii and started using alcohol and pills at age 15. After several relapses, Ivy went to a residential treatment program at The Camp Recovery Center, In Scotts Valley, and then straight to Gault House, in Santa Cruz.

Ivy, welcome.

Hi.

How did your addiction start?

I was born in Hawaii and raised there. At the age of about 12, my parents moved me from Oahu to the Big Island. I had a pretty nice childhood and great parents who loved me. At the age of about 14, I took my first drink. I remember exactly where I was. I was with a couple of friends and I was at a sleepover. One of my friends had an older sister and we got in the car with her and went to a party. I was offered a glass of white wine, which I took. I was a little nervous, I remember, but I drank it. I remember loving it. That's what I knew I wanted to do. I wanted more. There wasn't more and I was too shy to ask for more, but the feeling I got was like no other. I'm taken out of my normal mental state.

After that, I was about age 14, and I started hanging out with probably the wrong crowd and drinking more. Then it became an obsession. At 15 or 16, it was all about where I could find alcohol. Being too young to buy it, I was very creative and finding ways to get it, whether it was asking people in a parking lot how to get it or to buy it for me and my friends or dressing up as an older person and going into a store and just hoping for the best that someone would sell me alcohol. I would also take it out of my parents' cabinets. It became an obsession for me. I started doing cocaine around the age of 16. I had a cousin who I used to do it with. He was a little bit older than me. We would drink and do cocaine. He taught me how to get it. He would take me to this little corner in a little sleepy town in Hawaii called Hilo and he would say, "This is how you do it." We would wait for some random person, people to walk by, a lot of people who sold drugs were around there. He would say, "Can we buy a bag from you?" That's how we would get it.

I decided I wanted to do that on my own one night when he wasn't there. I went to that corner and there were a bunch of people down there. I got out of the car and I asked a couple people and they were like "What are you doing down here?" I was a 16-year-old girl. I said, "I'm trying to buy coke." There was a guy who was dressed pretty nicely in a leather jacket. He walked up to me and he was like "What are you doing here?" I said, "I'm looking to buy coke." He goes, "I'm the dealer." I said, "Can I get some?" He gave me a bag and he said, "Let's hang out." We hung out that night and for several nights after that. At that time, I was probably around 17. We started dating. He was quite a bit older than me. He was probably like 26 or 27 at that time. I started

274

dating him. He would take me to his house and I did a lot of cocaine with him. I was in and out of high school at this time, back and forth from my parents' house, and they were getting sick of me. I wasn't going to school, and all I wanted to do was hang out with this guy. Finally, I dropped out of high school and I told my parents goodbye and I left. They didn't know where I was. This was a bit before cell phones.

I basically was living off the grid. I'm probably eight miles from the main road or any other person. I'm down this very a creepy dirt road. I lived there with him for probably four or five months. My parents didn't know where I was. I did have a car that I had taken when I had left. He would take it from me and go and do his thing and he would be gone for days sometimes. I said, "The only thing that I want is to make sure that I have alcohol and drugs. You can use my car; just leave me some Top Ramen, cocaine, and alcohol, and I'll be good." I was basically stuck in this house and it was under construction. It was weird. I'm in the middle of nowhere by myself for days on end. I'm doing my drugs, waiting for him to come back to supply me, which he always would. It was never soon enough, but he would always come back.

Finally, I got in touch with my parents because I was sick of living like that. I felt like I needed help. He was abusive and I didn't know what I was doing. I was 17 at this time, so I got in touch with my parents. They were happy to hear from me and they had told me that they were moving from the Big Island to Oahu and if I wanted to go back and try to finish my senior year at a high school on Oahu. I said I would if my boyfriend, who I'll call Casey, could come with me. They agreed, so I moved into their home on Oahu and Casey came with me. He lived with me. He was probably 28 and I was 17. My parents were dealing with it because they were so freaked out that I had been gone for so long. He was abusive and would want to have sex with me and I had gotten to a point where I wasn't even attracted to him. He grossed me out, but as long as he would give me my drugs, I would be okay. I got pregnant in November of 1995 by Casey and my dad was super-pissed, but it was what it was. Casey went on to rob my parents' tenant of $20,000 worth of jewelry and did all of these very bad things and got kicked out of my parents' house. I was pregnant. I ended up graduating high school, which was a big thing for me at that time. I had my son in July of '96.

For the first six months, I didn't drink, and I didn't use. I knew that I was an alcoholic and an addict. I was scared to start again, because I knew that once I did, I wouldn't stop. I had this baby to raise. Slowly, but surely, I started drinking again; Casey was out of the picture by this point. I was living with my parents and I started to get into the party scene with my friends. My parents would watch my son and I would go be gone for weeks on end. At that time in my life, I was into Ecstasy. It was a big thing and I would do it many nights in a row, along with drinking. I was a blackout drinker. I'd drink as much as I could all the time until I would pass out. I was embarrassed when I would wake up but kept doing it.

This cycle started and did not end until recently. I went through life drinking, drinking, and drinking. My parents were helping me with my son, and at the age of about 25, I met a man who I ended up marrying. Here I am, I'm like "I'm finally getting it together. I'm finally figuring it out. I have a dad for my son." He was a heavy drinker, so we drink together a lot. We both were in the restaurant business and wine and alcohol was very glorified. That's what we did. We drank, but I was very functioning. I always held down a job by this point. My son was about seven. We got married and we moved to Lake Tahoe. My addiction started getting heavier and heavier now that I was in a place I had never lived. I didn't know anyone and I worked a lot. I would get off of work and start drinking until I passed out. I still was able to function.

In 2010, I got my first DUI. It was a day that my grandmother had died, and I felt like I was entitled to drink as much as I want. I got in the car to go buy a pack of cigarettes and I got a DUI. I spent the night in jail. That was my first time in jail. I got out and I was very traumatized. I couldn't believe that that had happened. I was scared, and I didn't know what I was going to do. That passed and my drinking continued to get heavier and heavier. My marriage was failing and a lot of that had to do with the drinking and being mean and waking up and having to apologize. In 2015, my son was going to graduate high school and I and my husband had decided that once he graduated we would separate and go our own ways.

I had met a man in February of 2015 who I had started seeing and I was still married. It was not the right thing to do, but I didn't care at that point. The alcohol had taken over and being with this new man wasn't an issue for me.

A couple of months later, I got diagnosed with breast cancer and I immediately freaked out. To me, it was almost like an invitation to keep drinking. It's like here I am. I'm the victim of cancer and I'm going to take this to another level. I got my doctor to prescribe me whatever I wanted because poor me. Here I am. I'm 36 years old and I have breast cancer. My doctors would give me what I wanted, which was mainly Oxycodone.

I had ended up having a double mastectomy and drank through the whole thing. I had a friend bring me wine in the hospital. I was there for three days and I said, "Please bring me some wine," and she did. I was on morphine, Oxycodone, kept drinking, and taking pills throughout the whole thing. They had told me that I had to have chemotherapy. To me, that was a huge thing. I was very angry at everyone around me and at myself. Why was this happening to me? I started my chemotherapy and got drunk one night and shaved all of my hair off. I woke up in the morning and I was bald. I knew it was going to fall out anyway, but it was a very traumatic experience to wake up with no hair. I continued to drink and use alcohol. I would go into these rages in a blackout and pull my wig off at dinner parties or in front of my parents' friends and throw it across the room and say, "Look at me. I'm a cancer victim." I played the cancer card. That's why I deserve to drink and use these pills and do them together as much as I could.

After several months of that, the chemotherapy ended, and I had to start radiation. I started the radiation and kept drinking. All of it started going to my head. Between the drugs and the chemotherapy, the radiation, the alcohol, and the pills, I started getting suicidal. My husband had left, but he was still around because he was trying to be the good guy. I started accusing him of cheating on me. It was an obsession. I would go to his work and sit outside drinking, popping my pills, and wait for him to come out with this imaginary girl. I was obsessed over it. When he would get home from work, it was always these huge blowouts of what he was doing and me throwing bottles across the room at him. How could he do this to me when I have cancer? One night, he had left, and I took a whole bottle of pills. I sent him a picture of the pills in my hand and I said, "Thanks a lot," or something close. As I took the picture, I took the pills and drank a bottle of Tequila and passed out.

I woke up in the mental hospital. I was trying to figure out what exactly happened. When he saw that picture, he had come, had gotten me, and the ambulance had come. I got put into ER and then the mental hospital for about four days. I begged my way out of the mental hospital because I wanted more alcohol. They didn't serve it there. I somehow convinced the doctors that I was fine, I needed more pills, and it was just because of the chemo brain. I kept saying, "I have chemo brain, so can I have more pills? I'll be totally fine." I remember the doctor saying, "Promise me," and I said, "I promise I will be fine." Within a week, I was back in the mental hospital. I'd done that whole thing over again, but I sent the picture to my best friend and said, "Thank you for being a best friend, but this is over." I took a picture and she called my parents. The same situation happened.

I woke up again in the mental hospital the next day, trying to figure out what the hell had happened. By this point, I was pretty brain-gone. My brain was not functioning at all, and I was extremely angry at the world and my family. Everyone tried to have like a counseling session, and I remember walking in with no hair in a gown, in a mental hospital, just screaming at them, "Look at me. What do you guys want from me? Look at what has happened to me. Just leave me alone. I don't want to have anything to do with you guys."

Looking at my mom crying and my sister crying and my husband who was beside himself, I got out of the hospital and literally packed my stuff up and left him for good. I moved into a little studio by myself and continued to drink and continued asking the doctors to give me pills. I had had several complications with my surgery and the radiation and my skin being able to hold the implant that they were trying to get in there. One particular instance was I had a roommate for a little while and he was a big drinker. We got in a huge fight in the middle of the night just over nothing important. I told him I was going to kill myself. I got up on the balcony and was going to jump. He grabbed me from behind and pulled me off of the balcony and squeezed my chest so hard that I passed out that night and I woke up in a pool of blood the next morning.

What had happened was he squeezed my chest so hard that the implant where the surgeon had sewed it up had popped up. The scar popped open and the implant was hanging out. I had to go to the doctor and he said, "What happened?" I said, "I don't know. I woke up in the middle of the night and my implant was exposed." He had to pull the implant out, so I was breast-less on one side for probably six months. During that six months, I was on and off work, between receiving Disability payments and not. I started randomly dating different guys. None of them were good guys. I always had the tendency to pick the ones who would drink with me and who could put up with me for at least a little while. Even ones who I didn't like or didn't like me or ones who I thought were the biggest alcoholics, thought I was a bigger alcoholic, and they couldn't handle my drinking. I knew at some point I was going to have to stop drinking, but I thought that that was far away. I was like one day I will stop drinking. This was 2016 or 2017. I was still on pills. I had the cops at the house a couple times for threatening to kill myself and telling people what had happened was that my disease was getting so bad that I didn't want to live. I was so depressed, and I had so much anxiety that the only thing that could mask it was the alcohol, and the alcohol was the problem that was ruining my life—a vicious circle, a downward spiral.

I was tossing me ability to function. I wanted to die. My parents tried to do a little intervention and I lost it. The thought of them trying to "control my life"—that was too much for me and I cut them off. I wouldn't talk to them because I felt like they were judging me. Did they know how much I had gone through? I ended up moving out of my place and into another little place. I started drinking more heavily than I had and it was always a blackout drunk. Everyone would bring these water bottles to work and I was working at a very high-end resort. In my water bottle would be vodka. I started drinking on the job. I started drinking during the day, putting Bailey's in my coffee, because that's normal. I'm drinking mimosas at the beach. Everything was an occasion for drinking, whether I worked or not. I worked in the restaurant business, so that would be a good reason to drink.

My new landlord and I became pretty close and she lived on the property. She kept saying to me, "Ivy, you have a very serious problem." I said, "No, I don't." She goes, "Look at all these bottles." I'm like, "I've had friends over." I didn't, but I didn't like it when people pointed that out to me. I had thought about possibly getting help, but I would have rather died. I figured I had three choices. One of my choices was dying. The second was getting sober, which was not an option. The third was living in the existence that I was living in.

How did you pay for your alcohol and your drugs? How low did you have to go?

I never stole. I worked hard, and I used men. I would have boyfriends and I would say to them, "Let's go get wine," and they would usually pay for that. Toward the end, I had this jar full of quarters that I had been keeping forever. I started not calling in sick to work, not being able to work, and using these quarters to buy my alcohol. I remember the week before I went into treatment, I was down to the last little bit of quarters there. I put it in the machine and I had enough for maybe one more bottle of wine. I would go to friends' houses. I would go to my sister's house, she lived down the road, and grab a bottle of wine from her house; just any way that I could get it.

What was the big spark that caused you to look for help to become clean and sober?

My last instance was I was dating this guy who I really liked. We had a lot of fun together and my son had come to visit me from California. I was in Hawaii; he was in college. He met the guy and I drank the whole entire time that he was there. I was wasted and both of them said something to me and I was like "Yeah, whatever." At this point, I was pretty far gone. I was drinking in the middle of the day in front of my son, which is something I hadn't done before. When he was growing up, I always somehow made sure it was at night. My son left early because he couldn't handle my drinking and this guy who I was dating, and I got into a huge fight with him and screamed at him.

I didn't even remember any of this until the next morning when I woke up sleeping on my lawn, looking for my phone. I found my phone and saw the texts and he said, "I don't want to have anything to do with you. I'm sick of this. I'm blocking you." He blocked me, which made me crazy. I tried to email him. I tried to do all these things and he wanted nothing to do with it. For me, I had to really look at myself and say, "My son left early." This guy who I really liked, but there had been a lot of them who I liked, had left, another person has left. Something clicked in me and I was like I'm going to end up an old lonely woman who's a drunk who no one wants to be around. That was my first thought after drinking super-heavily and using for 24 years that maybe it might be time.

What about your recovery? What is the real key to recovery for you?

For me, living here in this sober home has been huge. The support that I get here is amazing. As I walk in the door, there are always people who are like-minded. Everyone's in the same boat, trying to get sober and stay sober. Everyone's supportive, so that has been really helpful. I have a sponsor. I'm on my fifth step right now, and she's been amazing. She's helped me and talked me through all of this. I'm getting down to where this is all coming from. Also, I attend meetings. I did 90 meetings in 90 days. I'm trying to hit about five meetings per week. I'm now working two jobs, which I feel so fortunate to have.

What does your future look like?

I don't know. I'm just really excited about it. I feel like there are so many things I want to do, so many things I always wanted to do that I never felt like I could because I was so drunk all the time. How the heck would I be able to do those things? For me, I would love to get my yoga teacher-training license. That's something I've always wanted to do. I would love to meet someone maybe in recovery, maybe not, but have a healthy relationship and have meaningful relationships with everyone who I encounter. Being clear-headed for these last few months, it makes me realize how much time I have lost and how much I want to explore the world and books. I feel like I am a child who's reopened up into this world and looking for as much guidance and information as I can.

How confident are you about not drinking or using again?

I take one day at a time, every day. When I first was thinking about getting sober, one of my big things that I cried about, and I couldn't wrap my head around, was that I would never have fun again, that I was going to be this boring person and have to be in bed by 7:00 p.m. and never go to a restaurant again. All of that is not true, which is amazing to me. I do love to go to restaurants. There's never enough time during the day for me to do everything that I want to do.

As for confidence in not drinking, I take every day one step at a time. Sometimes it's just moment by moment, but it gets me through it.

One thing that I've found helpful is planning my day out. Waking up and thinking, I'm going to go to the gym, go to work, and then I plan the meetings that I want to go to. To be honest, I love going to the meetings. I go there, and I look around, and I'm like all of these people can do this. I can do this. I hear the stories and I feel not so alone.

As for confidence, I pray every day and I believe in my heart that I am going to get this, but it definitely is going to be something that I'm going to have to work for and something that is going to be with me for the rest of my life. I am having so much more fun and enjoying my sober life so much that I don't ever want to lose it.

Ivy, I want to thank you again for joining us here and sharing your story of addiction. To all of you, a big hug, and remember, today's the first day of the rest of your life.

4. JJ: Male, 41, Alcohol and Everything, Everywhere

JJ is a 41-year-old male from the San Francisco Bay Area. His drug of choice was alcohol, but he also had problems with everything else.

JJ, how are you doing?

I'm doing well.

Why don't you tell us how your addiction got started?

An important part of my story that informs why I ended up getting into drugs so early is that I was adopted. I don't remember any point in my life when I didn't know that. I assume there had to have been some point where I was able to understand it and was told, but I don't remember that happening. I remember growing up with that knowledge and feeling distinctly different from everyone around me. I've read a lot. I was an actor. I was in some commercials, TV, movies, and stuff. And when I was a little kid, I played the violin, a little guy. I didn't it in. I only had two, maybe three, friends all through elementary school. I pretty much always had my head buried in a book.

At the same time, I had a tremendous amount of rage inside of me. I can remember being as young as nine, 10, and getting enraged, blacking out, and knocking over bookshelves and punching through walls and things like that, seeing red. I fought a lot because I was a little guy. I was weird and nerdy, so I was a target. I was angry. I pushed back. When I got to high school, I had moved to Santa Cruz from Arizona. It was a new town. I was looking to try to start over. I joined the theater department there; I got into the school play and started making friends. Santa Cruz was a very different place from Tucson, Arizona, especially in 1992. It may be the only public high school in America where the stoners, metal heads, Goths, and freaks were at least in equal number to the jocks and the rich kids.

We had the whole front part of the school, the front lawn, and a little smoking corner across the street. The jocks had the quad, the back part of the school. I made friends with a guy in the theater department. He took a shine to me. I started hanging out with him. He was a popular, well-liked guy, had a lot of friends, and they all smoked weed. I started smoking weed. It didn't do anything for me the first several times I tried it. I do remember distinctly when it did work for me. I thought it was great. I started smoking weed every day. At the same time, I started attending school less and less. The first drug I ever did was LSD, before alcohol and before pot. It was this same friend who talked it up to me and he scored me and my neighbor, who was another nerdy weird kid. He played bass. I played guitar and we would jam on Misfits, Codes, and stuff in the garage. We took acid and went to the boardwalk. Neither of us had ever smoked any weed. We'd never had a beer.

You were totally drug-naive when you came here from Arizona?

Absolutely—I had a perception of alcohol as being what the jocks drank. I saw alcohol as being something that made you belligerent and aggressive, stupid, all of these things. Me and my friends, we didn't do that. We were the weird kids. We were in theater, sci-fi and fantasy. We were into expanding our minds. We would read Carlos Castaneda and Timothy Leary. Early on, I got into studying the drugs that I was taking while being on those drugs, taking them, and reading books about the way they worked chemically, even if I was too young to comprehend it. It was always fascinating to me.

For the first time in my life, I felt like I had friends, I felt like I belonged somewhere. Simultaneously, at home, my adoptive father had left. He was an abusive sociopath conman. He had bought a house on a credit card and lied and said that we were renting it. He didn't pay any taxes, lied, and said he had. He cut, ran, and filed bankruptcy. My mom is a single mother working full-time as a teacher, with $70,000 in debt. She had a complete nervous breakdown. I would wake up to go to the bathroom at 3:00 in the morning, and she'd be doing dishes and talking to herself. My father was the disciplinarian. With him gone, my mom had taken so much of a backseat that without his presence and the threat of violence that came with that, she had no authority over me. What she said meant nothing to me.

The extended family didn't exist. He took his extended

family with him. My mom's extended family—she grew up a poor white-trash girl and there weren't any family ties. I started developing simultaneously this family of choice, which revolved a lot around drug use, around psychedelic use. I started coming home less and less. I stopped going to school much. When I was a sophomore, my second semester, I went to one class one time; it was a choir and I showed up to that class because I got to play guitar. In the meantime, I was getting more and more into taking psychedelics on a regular basis. When I did go to school, I would go on psychedelics. I'm always smoking weed from the time I wake up until I go to sleep. I ended up getting kicked out of the house when I was 15. A friend of mine had a dad who was more like a buddy to him. He let him do whatever he wanted. He had his own separate wing in the house. He put me up for a month.

Did your mom know the progression that you were on in terms of drugs? Was she aware or did she see you're checking out or your behavior of not going to class? Did she know that drugs were right in there as part of what was going on?

My mom suspected that I was doing drugs. She accused me of being stoned on numerous occasions. I had a teacher who tried to intervene. She called her and told her that I was stoned. It was during after-hours play rehearsal and she showed up. It was one of the few times I hadn't smoked pot. I was gloriously indignant about it. The thing is, my mom never did any drugs. She's never smoked pot in her life, even though she was in college in the sixties. I don't understand it. She had a fiancé when she was young, in her early twenties, still in college, who died of a cocaine overdose. It scared her off of all drugs. While she suspected, she didn't know at that point, at least.

I ended up getting kicked out of the house. I was staying with a friend of mine and he drank. He had this different group of friends. They were not among my circle, but there was this Venn diagram overlap between his group, who we called the "Meatheads." They were metal heads and they drank. We were all hanging out one night. They were making fun of me for having never even tried alcohol. I was a little big man. But I'm a little guy. And I was ready to fight. I was ready to argue. I didn't let anyone smack me. I didn't let anyone put me down.

Basically, I got irritated into drinking because I wanted to show these guys up. I could consume Herculean quantities of weed and mushrooms. They had a stolen bottle of Kailua and a bottle of Seagram's Seven they had stolen. I chugged half of that fifth of Seagram's Seven. It's the first drink I ever drank. In the movies, you see people, they take their first drink, they gasp, and none of that; I chugged it. It burned, but I put a game face on. I drank some of that Kailua as a chaser. I got pretty drunk. I didn't throw up. I got the spins a bit. I ended up smoking a bowl later, which is when the spins came.

I liked it, but it wasn't like a light bulb went off revelation. Over the next few months, alcohol started to become more and more prominent. We were getting around 16 to 17.I was going to a lot of parties because I was homeless. I was always looking for somewhere to crash and parties were a great way to do that. I started drinking more frequently, maybe once a week or so. At that same time, I started liking pot and psychedelics. I'd had a bad trip and had another bad trip. I ended up in juvie. My mom kicked me out for a month, called the police, and reported me as a runaway. I've dropped by school. They came and they grabbed me and dragged me out of school in handcuffs in front of everybody, which boosted my reputation.

I don't say this to be self-aggrandizing, but to explain the culture I was living in at that time. This was in 1994, in Santa Cruz, California. The underclassmen, I found out from a girl I dated a couple of years later, had nicknamed me "JJ, King of the Druggies." I was a big man at that time, in those circles, the same volleyball captains who would drive by in their big raised-up pickup trucks and yell out, long hippie hair, thespian, etc. In geometry class later, he would tap me on the shoulder and say, "I'm sorry about that. I got to do that with my friend. Can you get me and my girlfriend some acid this weekend?" I would text them and double what I got it for.

I felt protected. I felt safe. I felt loved, all of these things that I had never felt at home. The alcohol started showing up more and I started doing the psychedelics less. When I was 17, I had somehow managed to test out of high school. I took the California High School Proficiency exam. It's a California-based GED-type certification. It's only good in California. You take it when you're 16. I took it a week after

I turned 16. I tested out. That first semester I was doing well. I fell in with this guy. He's another musician. We started hanging out. He introduced me to heroin. That was my first experience with the way that hard drugs can isolate you with other people in a way. It can create these insular, paranoid, little micro-cultures.

I dragged a couple of my friends into it. He had his girlfriend and her friend. There were six of us who were secretly doing heroin but still existing in this larger group of people where we were drinking and smoking weed and all that stuff. One of those other outer friends found out about my heroin usage and put together an intervention, my mom and a counselor and staff. They all tried to get me to go into treatment, but I had already decided I wasn't going to do heroin anymore. I did it six, eight times over the course of no less than a month. I woke up one morning and felt dirty. I felt like I don't want to be a heroin junkie. That's not what I want from my life.

I still had some level of aspirations. The music was always there through everything. I always thought that it was going to be what I was going to do. I was going to be a musician. I didn't go to treatment. My mom couldn't make me because she already kicked me out of the house. What could she withhold from me? After that heroin scare, I did straighten up a bit. I wasn't smoking weed anymore. I basically was drinking on the weekends at parties. Some years go by, and over the summer of 1996, four friends of mine all became meth dealers, like crank hit Santa Cruz like a tsunami breaking.

In August of 1996, I had been out of town for one month. I went on a long walkabout trek up and down the coast, hitchhiking and camping out. I got back and everyone I knew was on the crank. I was homeless again. I ended up doing it because that's who I was hanging out with where I ended up staying. I always had jobs, ever since I was 14, 15. I was always working. Even though I was homeless, I always had money. I would buy alcohol and later meth. People would let me stay at their place because I supplied the goods.

I had always maintained afoot in these two mirror worlds, I had my downtown druggie friends, I worked, and I had a lot of friends who were a little bit older than me who were at UCSC who didn't hang out downtown. I was able to keep it together, to keep what I was doing secret, until the meth hit. All of my more-together friends, they started doing meth too. Everyone I worked with was doing it. All the college kids were doing it. I ended up being the one who would run the meth, from the guys downtown to the college kids.

I had a house with eight college kids in it. That became my little sanctuary because I could go get an eight ball from my friends for them, bring it back, and hang out for a weekend. I could tell that things were starting to go bad. Everyone was tweaking up for so many nights, and rivalries were starting to form. These different dealers who had all been at least acquaintances started to become competitors as they got bigger and bigger and started dealing in the larger quantities and going for bigger scores.

One of the dealers hooked up with the girlfriend of one of the other ones, the guy who was the little Godfather of our

294

little area and started a little war. Things got crazy. I decided I was going to cut out. My best friend, who had been with me through all of this, had bounced off to this little town of Corvallis, Oregon, and would hang out with some friends of ours. He was calling me, trying to tell me to get up there and get off the crank. He had gotten off it. There wasn't any there, like it was a chill place. It's super-cheap up there. The two-bedroom house that we had was $400 or something.

I started putting my plans together. I had somehow managed to get a car at this point. I had a home. I had a job, so I was saving money. As it happens, I crashed the car, I lost the girl, I lost the place, all in the space of a few days. One of the dealers I knew, a bigger guy, was coming around, asking about me, because there had been some guys who I knew who had borrowed my car and used it to go burgle a place that I worked at. The detectives were calling me. In the meantime, this guy who was somehow involved in that was looking for me, trying to figure out if I was going to talk to the detectives. I tried to make sure I wasn't going to talk to detectives. Some people I was loosely associated with tied up, tortured, and murdered a man because he had molested one of them when he was a kid, and this led to police on a manhunt all the way to Florida. That was in '97 or something like that. It was international news. It was huge. I was associated with those people.

I left with nothing. I hopped on a Greyhound bus with a couple of $100 and went up to Oregon. It worked. I got clean in Oregon. We didn't drink because we didn't have any money. Coming from where I was coming from, where at that point, I was slamming glasses from San Francisco and getting a lot of pills, and pharmacies were getting knocked over. Crazy stuff was going on. It was coming from that, having some beers on the occasion where we had a few extra bucks. It felt pretty close to sobriety. I stayed up there for a little while, came back to Santa Cruz briefly, and went back up there. I ended up living with a couple of alcoholics, and that was the first time I discovered what it's like to wake up having panic attacks. You're so hungover, but still grabbed the bottle of bourbon that had a couple of shots in it at 9:00 in the morning, slammed it down, and kept that cycle going all day long.

I got out of there. Everyone I had known in Santa Cruz has either gotten killed, gone to jail, or ran. Santa Cruz was safe for me. This was a pattern I repeated all throughout my young life, as I would get in the shit and I would leave somewhere and think that by removing myself from the area where I was having the problems that everything would be okay again. I'd come back and there were different people. Things would be okay for a while, sometimes a few months, sometimes a few years. But eventually, a couple of years later, I would end up living with some people who were running meth again. This time, I was the one who was going to San Francisco and sitting in the closed dance studio underneath the cooks' apartment that he used for deals with a group of Vietnamese gangsters with machine guns, waiting to collect the bounty to take back and distribute in Santa Cruz.

I don't even know how that happened. I honestly don't. I was working and living with a guy who was a friend of mine, and both of us had been into all that. Then we weren't anymore. One night when we were all drinking way too much, somebody was like "Don't be funny. We could all do a line if we wanted to." We haven't touched meth in a couple of years. We could do it. It would be interesting. But it didn't work out. That house got crazy. I got run off at gunpoint. I was 21 at this point. I had loaded guns stuck in my face three different times all around meth. I had knives on my throat. I had left people on the ground unconscious and I don't know how that resolved.

I got this job, working 40 hours a week, but with the commute, it was more like 60 hours a week. I got in this band with a bunch of people who were older than me. We were still doing a lot of drinking and pills, but that was it. We went on tour. I went on this month-and-a-half-long tour. It was great. None of those guys did drugs. We drank like a fish and came back. Then 9/11 had happened a couple of weeks before we went on tour. That was weird. I got back to San Diego, and the place I was working at had gone out of business, everything had gone out of business. I moved to Austin, Texas. From there, for the next several years, I got back on track, as far as making the progress that a young man should be making at that age.

How old were you at that point?

I was 22. I went to Austin for a couple of years and learned how to live without drugs, with lots and lots of booze. I came back to Santa Cruz again briefly. I met a girl, moved to San Francisco, and I knew I'm getting married. I owned my own business. I sold that business for a tiny profit. I finally tracked my biological parents. That fundamentally changed something in me. The convergence of finding my biological parents, them wanting to be found, that being a good reunion and seeing how similar we were and also getting married. I had been a serial monogamous up to that point. Not even subconsciously—explicitly, I had a strong desire to try to reboot my life in that way. Find a girl, settle down, get married, maybe start a family. Clear the wreckage of my past and start over fresh, but I couldn't stop drinking.

After the '08 crash, I was 30. I was right where I felt like I should be at 30, which had always been a real big thing to me. Even with everything crazy that I had done when I was younger, I still wanted to live in that world of normal people. I don't know what else to call them. I wanted to have a career. I wanted to be someone who people will get introduced to their parents. I hadn't done anything to process the shame and resentment of my past. I was carrying all of that with me. That's why I was drinking so much; and even though my life was pretty good, I felt like a fraud.

Did you recognize that it was problematic, the amount of drinking you were doing?

Yeah. I'd started keeping it from my wife. We'd have wine at dinner. It was a running joke between us when I finally tried to get sober that first time; it took about two months to finally track down all the little airline bottles of vodka that

298

were in the car, rolling around every time you took a corner. It sounded like a slay jingling. I knew it was problematic. At that point, I had escalated to the point where I was working 70-hour weeks. I was drinking every minute of that. I was working at a startup company, 65-to- 70 hours a week, no days off. I was running a recording studio/label. I was playing in three bands and doing session work for five other bands because I play the violin. I was grinding myself in the ground and the only thing that kept me going was vodka.

My buddy who's still a big drinker, he tried pointing it out to me. He said, "When you get to where you're just drinking vodka, it's no different from a syringe. It's "medicine." I had to start drinking from the moment I woke up. I couldn't go an hour without a drink. When the economy collapsed, I lost my job. My whole industry vaporized overnight. My marriage started collapsing. I started having panic attacks that were bad enough that even the alcohol couldn't keep them down. At the time, I didn't understand that they were panic attacks. I didn't know that I had been having panic attacks for my entire adult life and probably a lot earlier than that. I thought that it was from the drink, withdrawing from the alcohol. I decided to stop drinking. Two days later, I was having seizures. My wife dragged me to a doctor and put me on a Klonopin prescription, put me on Seroquel, all these different meds. I was a zombie.

It had no point of reference. I started going to AA meetings, but I wasn't doing it for me. I was doing it because my wife had drawn a line in the sand. It was an ultimatum thing. She was making me do it. She got on any precedents.

Something happened where she stopped feeling anything. It seemed like she hated me. I was living with this woman who hated me, but I was committed to it, because I didn't want to be like my adoptive dad. I was going to stick it out because I made a commitment. My word is my bond and all this insane stuff. I was on all these crazy meds. I was occasionally still sneaking. If I have to show, I would play the Catalyst on New Year's Eve, getting up in front of 800 people and having never played a sober show in my life. But I was trying.

There were a lot of days when I was sober. They weren't good days. I had panic attacks all the time. I had never seen a real psychiatrist before. I was learning about anxiety and panic attacks, putting together how those two things went together. My wife started drinking again, but still insisting that I wasn't allowed to drink. When she and I met, she was puking by the end of every single night that I spent with her. She started running around with some other guy lying to me about it. She came home from this two-day conference thing. I knew that she had been with that dude. She lied to me on the phone. I called her out in person and she admitted to it.

She went to go stay at a friend's house and I left town for a week. When I got home, all my stuff was gone. She'd given away my dog to some stranger in Oakland, sold everything, except for my instruments, and left me at the end of the month, holding the bill on a $1,200-a-month place. I'm working at a record store at the time because it was the early days after the economic collapse, and making $10 an hour, I ended up staying with some friends. I'm on

Gabapentin and Klonopin, but I started drinking again, doing a little blow, anything because I was suicidal. I've never dealt with depression. I had never been sober long enough to realize that I even had an anxiety disorder.

I was getting all this stuff at the same time. I completely lost my mind. I stopped taking the Gabapentin, not realizing that all the side effects of that. I was still drinking heavily. I had a crazy psychotic episode. I burned bridges with all of my biological family, which I had met a few years earlier. Then I met a woman who was awesome, caring, wanting to go to school be a nurse, got me to quit drinking, by not telling me I had to quit drinking, but by being sad that I was punishing myself. I got it. She didn't make me go to meetings or anything. She said that she couldn't be with me if I was going to be out-of-control drunk all the time.

For those three-and-a-half years, I started rebuilding myself as a normal citizen. I became part of the world again. We moved to Seattle, had some good jobs. I would still drink at any of the types of occasions that people would drink at and sometimes at home, but I was careful not to get drunk. Every drink I had, every drink I didn't have, and every moment of the day, I was aware of the presence of alcohol in the world. I was counting the drinks. I was spacing out the time. I've seen my biological dad. I've seen him do it. He's been a functioning alcoholic since he was in his twenties because he has these rules. As my buddy said, here are these rules.

He doesn't start drinking until 4:00. I see him at 3:55 and he's standing there in the kitchen staring at the liquor cabinet, the obsession. I could not shake that. Eventually, we split up amicably because we both realized that I was doing the thing where I got with someone who helped me. I ended up in the hospital early in our relationship because I was punishing my liver so bad. I wasn't able to keep food down. I didn't eat for three days because everything I tried to put in my stomach came right back out. I was told that I was going to die if I did not stop drinking now. I was doing that thing where I was with a woman who I felt like it saved my life. I went with her up to Seattle, left everything I had behind, so she can go to nursing school, and I supported her as much as I could through that.

She was doing 70-hour weeks. I did the laundry. I'd cook and stuff like that. I got her through nursing school. We reached this point where it's like "I need to go be on my own." I've not been single for more than nine consecutive months since I was 16 years old. At this point, I was 35, 36. She's an amazing person. I still love her with all my heart. I still consider her one of my best friends. She got it and she didn't want it. She was not willing to be on a pedestal to be my savior. We had conversations about that. She was uncomfortable with that aspect of our relationship. I got it. I went back home to Santa Cruz. I was still on a real good streak. I was working full-time at Trader Joe's. I picked up a second job doing catering, bartending. I was going to school full-time. I was taking honors classes. I had a 3.8 GPA. I was running.

Anytime I thought about getting high or getting drunk, I would throw on my running shoes and go seven miles, eight miles. I did run 35 miles a week. I rode my bike to Cabrillo and back. It was 40 miles a week of that. I was sleeping maybe three or four hours at night because I couldn't. I had taken my addictions, that obsession and I moved it over onto things. On paper individually, all these things look fantastic. Everyone's clapping me on the back saying, "You're killing it. You're doing good." I was even able to buy a six-pack, bring it home, have a beer, and let it sit in the refrigerator. That was one of my long-term goals for my life when I was in my early twenties. I want to have a liquor cabinet. I want there to be liquor in it. Tomorrow there's still booze in there. It was a fantasy. I was doing it because I was putting all that obsession into all those other things I was doing.

I've had similar thoughts before. You and I, we can't necessarily know, certainly not subjectively, but what it's like to be a normal person. The mere fact that, as you say, being able to have something like that is a fantasy, or the similar thoughts that I've had that aren't normal—that a normal person, it's not even a thought, It's like "I'll pick up a bottle or do a little coke in the night out with friends or whatever." They don't think about the next day. It's not some constant thing. It's not the goal of being able to moderate because moderation comes naturally. One time I went through treatment and I had already been a bunch of times and I was so certain I can handle drinking. I've never had a problem with alcohol. I'm going to do it. It's like "Why does it matter? If I was so focused on that, shouldn't I have realized that the mere fact that I'm focused on it is itself the problem?" You're here. You must have reached some clarity around that at some point?

I never understood that "normies" don't have that obsession. I didn't understand that until I went to treatment. I did not get it. Part of that is because I didn't know anyone like that. I didn't because anyone like that fell away from my group of friends, even the ones who were also killing it, keeping their lives together and stuff like that. If I talked to them about booze; they were nervous about it. They had concerns. They understood that it was problematic for them. They're at points where they were, for whatever reason, handling that well and maybe that will continue. Maybe it won't. I don't know. This is something that I go around with myself, especially after going through treatment.

I believe that the same affliction, genetic cork that is responsible for an addictive personality, is linked to other positive qualities, as well like to creativity. Obsession can manifest as an intellectual curiosity and a passion for passion. By and large, most of the addicts who I've known when not in the thralls of active addiction had been passionate, creative people. Yet I'm a little tentative around that idea because I can see how that could also be me trying to get myself a pass a little bit or trying to soften how destructive addiction is.

You could go the opposite way with it too, though. It's something that I frequently say that the addiction is part of the human condition and that everybody is an addict in some form or another. Some of us take it way earlier in-depth than others, even if it's not to substances, to behaviors of some sort, shopping, sex, gambling. Even

304

in smaller things like television or social media, it's pervasive across society. If you called out a so-called normal person who maybe spends a few hours a day on Facebook or whatever, they're not going to see it as an addiction because it doesn't affect their lives the way drugs have affected yours, for example.

I agree with you; I know what you're saying. I don't recognize that there's at least an element of that, particularly in creative people or intelligent people.

There was a counselor who came in to do classes at Janus Recovery Center that I was at who explained addiction in a way that stuck with me. The Big Book talks about alcoholism as an allergy, which I always thought as off the mark. It's like almost the thirties, how quaint. She explained how, for any substance, let's take alcohol—alcohol does have a chemical hook. We know pretty much that the chemical hook in and of itself is not the most important driver of addiction. Every person on Earth has a threshold, a certain amount of alcohol they can consume before they crossed this threshold into addiction. Once that switch has been flipped, they are an addict. That's the same way that an allergist explained allergies to me, is that we're all allergic to everything that causes the allergic reaction.

We have different levels of histamine resistance basically. You can be a cat lover for your whole life. When you're 81 years old, you could wake up one morning and be horribly allergic to cats because you've been bombarded by these allergens for so long. It's broken down your resistance the same way with alcohol. It's something she didn't touch on that I see is different in people like me, the trash can thing. It's not like I drank enough alcohol that I triggered an addiction. I've been addicted to quieting the inner voice, anything to take me out of my normal state of being, which for most of my life has been one of fear and shame. They had ruled the overwhelming majority of my life, starting from when I was young.

What happened to get you into treatment that first time?

When I was doing all that stuff, working those two jobs and going to school, I don't know, I had a collapse; I collapsed at work. I got ill. It was the symptoms. It was like I had a brain tumor. I had Nystagmus. My balance was messed up. My skin was going crazy. I couldn't digest. I couldn't eat anything. I got down to 119 pounds. I was walking with a cane. Eventually, they figured out that there were these polyps in my intestines that were building white blood cells and dumping them into my system, which were attacking my brain and other organs. They removed them. That's not happening. There was still damage, so I had to go to two years of neuro-physical therapy because my memory had been destroyed. It was all kinds of crazy things like that.

I wasn't able to work obviously during that time. I mentioned earlier that I've worked since I was 14. I worked through homelessness, drug addiction, everything. I've been very self-reliant my entire life and not being able to support myself having to lean on the government until that stopped. It made me suicidal. I became extremely depressed, and that's not something that I grew up with. I didn't have any coping skills for it. I was having seizures from this weird autoimmune thing. I've been put on Klonopin again. I was on an antidepressant. I was on six different medications. I felt old and useless and that my life was over. I had missed the opportunity to have a life. It was too late for me. There was no point in my existence, but I wasn't selfish enough to kill myself.

I could not bear doing that to my family, my adoptive mom, who was the one who was taking care of me at the time, in particular. I wanted to annihilate my consciousness. It was the first time that my drinking was motivated solely by crushing despair and a desire to die. I was still on Klonopin, so I was blacking out. I had no idea what happened. One of those times, I woke up in a jail cell and that sucked. I ended up stuck in there over the weekend because I got arrested on a Friday. I did not want to repeat that experience. I became committed to getting sober. I had hit bottom. The jail cell was finally after the divorce, after everything else that had happened in my life, and I finally plowed through all those false bottoms and hit bedrock.

A switch was flipped and I wanted to get sober, but I was still suicidal and massively depressed, even more so now, as I was addicted and on Klonopin, which is booze in a pill with all the fun parts sucked out of it. I tried. I committed. I went to meetings. I wanted to be sober, but I would get so overwhelmed by this crushing depression that I had chain panic attacks, one after another. Every few months, I couldn't hack it. I would drink like a whole bottle of vodka and immediately black out. It's not a good experience, blacking out, and I was brutally ill because the combination of Klonopin, antidepressants, and liquor—it's not good; It doesn't make you feel well.

The third time that happened, I was still living on my mom's couch because I hadn't been able to support myself, and I briefly got a job at a grocery outlet, but I was still too frail and also the Klonopin. I couldn't do the work. I wasn't physically strong enough. That made things even worse. I had business cards I made for myself when I was in my early-twenties that said, "I can do that." That was my motto. I've worked jobs from shoveling manure, on a goat farm, to nonprofits, working with at-risk youth, to film production. I've done everything outside of the trades. To not physically be able to support myself, it destroyed me. There was nothing left.

I ended up going into treatment. A sense in my mind, how I talked to myself and to go into new treatment was to get off Klonopin because I talked to my doctor about getting off it. He said it would take a year to safely taper off the amount I've been taking it for as long as I had. He was also the medical director at Janus. He may have been partially helping me convince myself that it was okay to go to treatment. I went for that. I went through a month-long brutal detox from that. I had a couple of seizures, left, and I didn't listen when they were talking about PAWS, the Post-Acute Withdrawal Syndrome.

I got a job. I got into a sober house. I was doing well for a couple of weeks when that post-acute withdrawal hit. I stopped sleeping; I started having crazy panic attacks. I couldn't sleep. I went totally insane. I ended up relapsing; I didn't want to. I just couldn't sleep; I couldn't think. I've talked to people who worked with me and around me at that time. They were convinced that I was messed up on some heavy crap before I relapsed. I was absolutely nuts with sleep deprivation and anxiety. I went back to Janus for another month, got on this amazing medication, Remeron, which helps with your circadian rhythms. It doesn't knock you out and make you feel stupid the next day. It allows me to sleep like a normal human.

The first week that I was in Janus, I was awake for 80 consecutive hours, no caffeine, nothing. I did not sleep for three-plus days. I got on the Remeron, and I started having regular restorative sleep every single night. The panic attacks went away. I thought back on it. I remember being in third grade and waiting for the sounds of everyone going to sleep, so I could get up and go read or whatever. I've never been able to sleep my entire life. I'd sleep maybe one night, five hours the next day, three, and then not at all. There was a 40-hour period that I was contiguously awake for basically every week or two as far back as I can remember.

Getting regular restorative sleep and getting off Klonopin and getting off the antidepressants, I feel like a totally new person. I'm physically healthy, strong enough to work. Those basic things have become the bedrock of my sobriety. I'm able to go to shows now. The first show I went to after I got out of treatment the last time, I didn't even notice I was in a bar for the first hour that I was there until I saw someone next to me holding a beer, and I was like "That's what they do here." The obsession, at least in the last however many days I've been here, for several months, the obsession is not there anymore. I attribute it to sleeping at least seven hours every night, eating well, eating when your body needs food, and getting regular exercise, but not like the excessive exercise I was doing, but doing therapy and the step work, processing all the shame and resentment that had driven a lot of my behavior. My program is a simple one because I've been missing these fundamental things, like sleep and food. I never ate either, for a great deal of my life.

What's your hope or plans for the future?

I want to be able to support myself. If I had a loftier goal, it would be to enjoy my work, to have work that is meaningful to me. I've found a new job and I like it. I see opportunities and to have my life be meaningful in some small way—nothing more grandiose than that. I sincerely don't think I'll ever own a house. And I pray to God I never get married again.

If you had any advice for somebody who's maybe dealt with some similar things to yourself and is considering getting into treatment or considering this lifestyle change, what might that be for them?

I would say that if you haven't totally blown your life up yet and you think you have a problem, why don't you try not picking up whatever it is that you're picking up? Give yourself 30 days. It's amazing to me how many people can't do 30 days. It's also amazing what a dramatic change you'll see in that short period of time. At the end of that 30 days, it's not like booze will be outlawed a month from now. Try, and if you have blown up your life and you sincerely need to make a change, but you don't know how, be willing to change everything in your life. Even down to wearing clothes you would never normally wear, change everything and be willing to let things go. You may have to move. It's worth it.

Considering you did a lot of your drug use here in Santa Cruz, I did almost all of mine here and we're both here and we are both sober. I would say it's certainly possible to get and stay sober where you used. I like the idea of somebody, if they don't know whether or not they have a problem, give them a month. Even if they're able to stay sober for that month, I think that if their mind is going to focus in on that thirtieth day and like "When do I get to do after that?"That's addiction right there.

Thank you so much, JJ. Thanks to all our readers. We wish you to stay sober and be happy.

5. Kendra, Female, 34, Heroin and Homelessness

Kendra is a 34-year-old woman who suffered a back injury in a car accident in her teenage years. This caused chronic back pain, and Kendra abused the prescription pain pills. When the pain pills got too expensive, Kendra switched to heroin, and homelessness followed. Kendra attempted recovery several times, but relapsed several times. Kendra wants to be a good mother to her seven-year-old son and this is part of her motivation to find the recovery lifestyle.

Kendra, hello. I know you are feeling nervous. Thank you for being here to share you story of addiction. How did your addiction start?

Around my mid-twenties or so, I discovered pain pills and they gave me relief from the chronic back pain I had been experiencing since a car accident as a teenager. That was the beginning of the road. It was an instant way to get relief from the back pain that I have had for so many years. Fairly quickly, I began to build up a tolerance. I went on to need stronger pain pills, which eventually led to switching from pain pills to heroin. I was eventually using heroin. That started around age 24 or 25. That was when my addiction took over my life. Throughout my addiction, I made quite a few attempts at getting clean and sober. I've been to a couple of different recovery programs over the course of the last eight years or so. I have had a lot of clean time, but quite a few relapses as well. I was very blessed with the birth of my son. I had a son about seven years ago, and ever since then, I've had a strong desire to be able to get clean and be healthy for him and be there for him.

Tell me about some of the experiences you had during your drug using.

I've used drugs when I had money to spend on drugs. I've used drugs when I was flat broke and did not have money to spend on drugs. Not having the money to support a drug habit is a very quick way to wind up doing things you never thought you would do, doing things you know are just not you. You know they're not you, but you know there's just something inside you that overpowers that voice and tells you that you need to do whatever you need to do to be able to continue to feed that addiction. I've done a lot of things that I'm not proud of, stealing food and stealing clothes when I needed them. I have also spent a short amount of time homeless, without a home as a result of my addiction, my disease.

When you're down to the bare nothing, your number-one priority when I'm active in my disease is to continue to feed that addiction, but then there are also the essentials of life, like food, clothes, staying warm, and all that. Those are the times when I have been homeless or down and out. I have shut people out of my life who are good people, positive people to have in my life, and traded that out for the people who I've needed to associate with throughout my addiction. Those times definitely were the times where I found myself going to those low places and doing those things that none of us are proud of.

When I was homeless, I've couch-surfed. I've stayed with friends and I've also physically been out on the streets with literally nowhere to go at night. It is a dark place to be in. You wind up resorting to survival instincts and survival methods, things that are going to get you what you need to survive. For example, if I was hungry, I would have to steal my food from a grocery store because I didn't have money to buy it. If I was cold and didn't have money to do laundry, I might have to steal warmer clothes. At the time, it can be easy to justify that behavior, because you do feel like you need it and you feel like you deserve those things like everyone else deserves them. It can be very hard to separate in your head the right from the wrong or whether it's acceptable for you to be doing these actions. It's just a sad era right now with what drugs have done in this community and how many people have been left homeless and penniless because of drugs. It's very sad.

How did you administer your drugs?

I started with the pills and that was oral administration. After I had gone from pills to using heroin; I started out smoking heroin. That's how I was introduced to it and how I would do it. I told myself, as I know many people have told themselves, I would never ever cross that line of going to IV drug use. The day did come where I did cross that line and then I became an IV drug user. I did wind up shooting heroin.

When you're out there shooting heroin, what did you do? Where did you live when you were on the streets and where did you get your money?

As far as where I actually lived, the choices were slim. There were nights I tried to curl up on a bench. My main memory of my period where I was homeless and out there with no roof over my head was that I got very little sleep, to be honest, a couple hours or an hour here and there. It was just staying up until my body could no longer stay up. Then I would get as much sleep as I needed and keep going.

What caused you to turn away from drugs and return to recovery?

This time around, I feel that I hit an emotional bottom more than anything else. I have unfortunately put myself in the hospital a couple times because of this disease and just how gnarly it can be and how much it can take from your body. Since my last relapse and then getting clean, I didn't drive myself into the ground physically. I just hit a point where I no longer wanted to live life the way I needed to live life when I was using. They speak in the program about the incomprehensible demoralization and I've heard it plenty of times before, but this has been a point where I'm looking back and I'm realizing I hit that point. I hit that incomprehensible demoralization. If I looked in the mirror, I didn't know who I was looking back at and I don't want that. I don't want that for myself and I certainly don't want that for my son. I want him to have a healthy, thriving mother who can be there for him.

What did your early recovery days look like?

I've had several very solid attempts at getting clean that have been successful. I would eventually, at some point, wind up relapsing again. I'm lucky to have found a wonderful sponsor. She is truly a lifesaver in my eyes and in my heart. I'm working with her and giving it my all. I'm giving 110 percent and she's taking me through the steps. She's helping me get through things that come up and there might be times in the past where I wouldn't have been able to handle the situation and would have wanted to just shut my eyes and escape and wind up relapsing because of it. I've been making a huge effort to lean into her, lean into the program. The rooms of Alcoholics Anonymous and Narcotics Anonymous have been wonderful to me. Everybody has been incredibly loving, accepting, and understanding. I hear things in those rooms that help me keep going. They help, whether it's reminding me what it's like to be in the disease or reminding me that there are other people who have gone through what I've gone through or whatever it is, it's a real feeling in the program of togetherness and we need one another. I want to be there for other people and help others get through this.

What is your opinion of this 12-Step Program?

Personally, I am grateful to have found this program that revolves on the 12 Steps because I feel like I get to go walk through those steps and then I drop them into my life to be a better person and find growth and development as long as I have that desire. I personally think that every human being could use the 12 Steps, whether they're an addict or not. We're lucky in this program to have the 12 Steps. They're a true aid in helping somebody develop the tools they may not have to get through life and be a contributing member of society and to learn to love myself again. That's one thing I am quite confident I'm going to gain from doing these steps. I'm going to connect with myself or reintroduce myself to me, but a version of myself that I love and that I know I am and can be.

Kendra, what else do you think works in recovery?

It is a very simple set of guidelines or suggestions. It's the willingness to take any suggestion, even if it's not every suggestion that you're given, especially by our sponsor or by other members in the program who you might look up to or might be living a life that resembles something you want to live. It's important to be willing. Willingness is a big one in my book.

What does your future look like to you?

My future looks very positive. My main priority is making sure that I get as healthy as I can get emotionally, spiritually, mentally, and physically, so I can be there for my son. I want to be there for anything he might need or want from me. I'm blessed to have him. He's an amazing kid and I want to give him the mother he deserves.

Thank you so much. Is there anything else you'd like to add?

I could not be more grateful at the moment. I could not feel more gratitude for what I've already been given in recovery and sobriety. If anybody out there is feeling like they're absolutely at the lowest point they can be at, or that there's nobody out there who could possibly understand how they feel and what they're going through, and the hopelessness they might be feeling, I want to say that the recovery lifestyle does exist. There are people who can help you through this thing; it truly is out there. You just have to be willing to take that first little step to ask for the help. There are many people in recovery who want to help you to overcome your addiction.

Kendra, thank you.

You are very welcome.

6. Michelle: Female, 29, Sexual Molestation & Loads of Alcohol

Michelle is 29-year-old woman. Her parents did not provide a good environment for her and her siblings growing up. When Michelle was 11, her uncle sexually molested her and used guilt to keep her quiet. Michelle has worked her way up within the restaurant industry, from a hostess to restaurant manager. She has made many of the mistakes that are commonly made within a management position, such as wanting to be liked, socializing with employees, drinking with employees, and dating employees. Michelle has more than $40,000 dollars in student loan debt. Michelle's honesty in discussing her journey into alcoholism is exceptional. She has a positive attitude that shows the miracle of the human spirit.

Welcome to the interview, Michelle.

Thank you.

How did your addiction start?

I'm going to go all the way back for this one. We're going to talk about my parents mostly because I fully believe that addiction is much more than who we are as people. It was our environment. It's the people who raised us. It's all of that. A lot of people you'll hear say that it wasn't. I don't want to blame anything, but these things have effects on us for sure.

I was born to two parents who were alcoholics. They also had a drug addiction. What that drug of choice was I do not know. I was born in Arizona, but I know nothing about that state, because we moved directly after. We moved all the time. We moved from Arizona to California to Barstow, California. We were all over. Whenever they ran out of money, we were on to the next place. At the time, I had five siblings. We had a large family. I lived with them until I was about four years old. I don't know if you've ever been to Barstow. It's not a great city to drive through. It has a huge drug problem, so they found their place in it. I remember many things where it was not the life that a kid is supposed to have.

I remember my biological mother asking my sister and me to go to the local liquor store and go steal some Twinkies and Ho Hos for her. I remember the police barging into our house because my dad was getting arrested for something. We were free-range kids. We took care of ourselves. We took care of each other. We were always getting into trouble and we had nobody there to tell us any different because they were busy with their own addiction. I can remember people coming in and out of our apartment. We moved many times, even within Barstow. We had a house at first, but they couldn't afford it after a while. We had an apartment and then we were living in a motel. We would downgrade as their addiction got worse. I didn't know that as a kid, but I can see that now as an adult. The downgrade is a direct result of them getting deeper into their addiction. When I was about three, my oldest half-brother and sister were taken by their dad. They left and then it was the four of us. It was my older brother, my older sister, me, and my younger sister.

There came a point where my parents couldn't take care of us anymore. My grandparents took us. My grandparents were my maternal grandmother and her second husband. He wasn't technically my biological grandfather. I had never met my biological grandfather, so he was the only grandpa I knew. We moved in with them in Southern California. It was good, but there was always something missing when you don't grow up with your biological parents. They always have a parent day at school. They always ask you to do a little tree thing as a project for school and you can't do that. It's a little bit of a bummer, but I know that my grandparents tried as hard as they could. My grandfather was always active in my school life. They did the best that they could. When I was 10, my grandmother developed breast cancer and spine cancer. She passed away. We had her in hospice care in our house and I was there the day she died. The house was in her name. We couldn't stay there anymore. My grandpa took all four of us, my older brother, older sister, younger sister, and me to Northern California to his daughter and her husband's house. They already had a kid. They had a kid who was outside the house. They had five dogs. His daughter's husband was in a wheelchair. There is not enough space for all of the kids and stuff.

When we moved up there, it was free-rein again. There were so many kids, they didn't have enough energy and time to watch all of us. We were outside and doing our own thing, which was fine, I'm not going to lie. I have some good memories of rollerblading outside, biking to the grocery store, and all that good stuff. It wasn't all bad for sure, but there were definitely not enough adults watching over the children. Probably in about August of 2000, my maternal aunt and her husband came and took my older sister because they wanted to be able to help out. They knew they could adopt, but they wanted to start with one, because they didn't have any children of their own. They took my sister and that went pretty well. They had her for a couple of months, and then it was me, my older brother, and my younger sister. It was at that time that my grandpa's daughter's husband molested me. I was 11 at the time. It started out super-innocently. All the kids were like "Let's give each other massages or whatever," and then everyone left, and it was just me and him. He was like "Why don't I give you a massage?"

I knew stuff wasn't right when he started to move lower and lower and then it all happened quickly and I felt numb. He asked me if he could hold me after and I wanted to scream, "No, you can't. You can't touch me anymore," but I was 11. I sat there in shock and I'd let him. He's in a wheelchair. There was a part of me that was always like why didn't you run? But it didn't make sense. The next day, we're doing some yard work or whatever. He pulls me aside and he goes, "You can't tell grandpa. You can't tell my wife. If you do, I'll go to jail and you'll upset everybody. You're going to break up the family," putting it on me because it would be my fault and not him taking responsibility for his actions. That secret ended up carrying with me for a long time.

In about December of 2000, my aunt and uncle came

back. They were like "We can take another kid. We'd be happy to." They're pretty well off. They both went to college and have nice jobs. They came back, gathered me up, and took me with them. We ended up moving into a house in Northern California because they got a job up there. What originally started out with six kids, with my two half-siblings, my older brother, my older sister, my younger sister and I, ended up being just me and my sister, with my aunt and uncle. My older brother and my younger sister moved back to Barstow with my biological parents somehow. They came and got custody of them. Meanwhile, my aunt and uncle got custody of me and my sister. My sister and I are much closer than any of the other siblings in my family.

We moved into Northern California. I was 11-and-a-half. I haven't been surrounded by addiction and violence my whole life, but I have been put into weird situations that have in turn made me a strange type of person. I didn't learn to deal with things the way normal people deal with everything else. When I moved in with them, they had never had kids before. They had to figure it out as they went. They would come up with creative punishments, which were always weird. If I didn't turn in a homework assignment, I would have a TEA SPOT, which stood for "Take Everything Away for a Short Period of Time." From Friday night until Monday morning, I would have to sit upstairs in this little office area. I wasn't allowed to talk to anyone. I wasn't allowed to read anything. I wasn't allowed to do any homework. I had to sit there by myself for two-and-a-half days. You couldn't do anything. You had to sit there for two-and-a-half days not talking to anyone. Lunch and dinner was a peanut butter bagel and water. Breakfast was Cheerios and a glass of milk. Monday morning, you finally got to go back to school. Those always pissed me off because it always seemed an overreaction to everything that was like a five-point homework assignment and I get an entire weekend taken away from me. On the other hand, I could have done the homework assignment and not gotten it. Mentally going through a TEA SPOT was not great.

It was mentally challenging to sit there by myself with nothing to entertain me for two-and-a-half days. Mind you, I didn't just have one of these. I had a whole summer of them once. I sit by myself at the table not talking to anyone. If I was a minute late downstairs to be ready, I had to pay this glass pumpkin $20. If I didn't do a chore on time, I had to pay the pumpkin. They did the best they could. When I graduated, all that money in the pumpkin was given back to me. I've had a job since I was 14. To have the little money I'm making be put into this thing, it's a punishment. I get the money back so it's not punishment? The same thing goes for the TEA SPOTS. I could have done the homework assignments, but I was like every other kid. I'm going to skip a couple of assignments. I am forever grateful to my aunt and uncle for taking me out of a situation that could have continued to be horrible. I don't know what my grandpa's daughter's husband would have continued to do. Who knows? I could have gone back with my biological parents, which also doesn't seem healthy.

Even though things were weird and I still didn't learn to be normal, which I always desperately wanted, I'm grateful to them and the opportunities that they've given me. I would not be who I am now without them. That's all I wanted. When I was in high school, you still have those stupid homework assignments where you're like "Tell us about your parents. Tell us about your grandparents. Tell us where you came from." I don't know. We had this rule when I was in high school: Don't ask questions. I don't know anything about anything. You're not allowed to ask questions. My aunt does not like her stepdad. He's passed away, but we weren't allowed to talk about him. Even though he was my grandpa, you weren't allowed to talk about him. I know nothing about him. I don't know anything about my grandma because we weren't allowed to talk about her either. My aunt doesn't talk to her sister, my mom, at all. I don't know why we're not allowed to talk about it. I'm in this cave of mystery where I know nothing because I'm not allowed to talk about it.

Finally, I turn 18. All I wanted was to be normal. I've never been normal my entire life. I had the addicted biological parents. I lived with my grandparents. Then I lived with my aunt and uncle. I didn't have the key to my house the entire time I was in high school. I'd sit on my porch no matter if it was raining. It didn't matter how hot or cold it was. I'd sit there and wait until both of them got home because I took my bike one time without permission and got hit by a car. I ended up losing the key to the house because of that. We're talking several years of high school and the entire eighth grade, many years without the key to the house.

When I say things weren't normal, they definitely weren't normal. We had weird punishments. We had a no-talking rule. I don't know anything about where I come from or anything like that. I don't know anybody on my biological dad's side. When you talk about medical history, nothing, I have no idea. That's something important to know. I turned 18 and I got accepted into SDSU. I was 18 at the time. From this point forward, I will call my aunt and my uncle my mom and dad because that's who to me are my mom and dad. My dad told me, "Don't go to college if you're not ready," but at the time that didn't make sense to me. I was like "That's what you do. You graduate high school, then you go to college." Fortunately, because of my weird family history, I was able to get good financial aid because they want your biological parents' financial income and I hadn't talked to them since I was four. They didn't reach out to me to be like "How's it going?"

The one time that my biological mother reached out to me was via Facebook and it was a message. She goes, "How's it going?" I haven't talked to this woman since I was four. The reason I'm not with her is that she was a drug addict and alcoholic and that's the first thing you have to say to me? I never messaged her back. I was like ""I'm good." I got good financially because I don't talk to my parents. I don't know what their income looks like. Since my aunt and uncle are technically only my guardians, I don't have to put them as my financial guarantors. I got good financial aid, which was bad because I went to San Diego and I went to zero classes. Not a single one. All of them were gone. I spent that money on rent and alcohol. I got down there and I couldn't get into a dorm. A dorm probably would have been better because I would have been surrounded by people. Instead, I got an apartment where I had the liberty to throw parties and live a life outside of school, which is probably not what I should have been doing. My dad was completely right. I should not have gone to college if I wasn't ready. Now, I know what that means. I'm like "I should have waited. I should have saved the money because student loans are horrible."

That started my drinking career. I remember starting to drink because I wanted to feel normal and I never have. Even in recovery, I still don't feel normal, but I embrace it now. The only time I could feel everyone likes who I am is when I was drinking. When I was drinking, I was grade A. Everybody loved me. I didn't have to double-think myself. I didn't have to over-think how I was interacting with people because I don't know why it was such a big deal to me when I was 18. It killed me that people thought I was weird and I can't tell you how many times people are like "Michelle, you're so weird," and that killed me. Being called weird killed me. I could see what they're talking about, and not in weird circumstances and stuff. In situations, I get weird. I'll look at something, play with something, or do something that's a little bit weird and not what normal people would do.

I like that it makes me unique. I'm a little weird. I'm a little goofy, but it's cool. That's who I am. When I was 18, I couldn't stand that. I had a way out. I could drink alcohol. I'm not sure why I was obsessed with the idea of whiskey, but I was. Whiskey is what I went for. I tried vodka. I hated it. I used to chase raspberry vodka with a bagel so that I could take more shots. I would do that super-nerdy thing where you keep track on your wrist of how many shots you do and then you go, "I totally blacked out and I didn't keep track of all of them. I took way more than this." It's loser stuff, but it seemed super- cool when you're 18.

I ended up living in that apartment for a year. I have to say when I was sober I still didn't feel comfortable in my own skin. I was always looking for acceptance. I was always looking for attention. I always wanted to feel loved. I was far away from my sister, my aunt and uncle. I went to college with my best friend, but she ended up finding her group of people. At first, I hung out with her, but she had found her group of people. I wasn't mad at her for it, but they weren't my group of people. They weren't my friends. I was the hanger-on and they were her group of friends. At some point, I isolated myself and stayed at the house. Sometimes I can't even explain the decisions I made. I never got a job while I was there because I was living off of financial aid until March.

I ended up getting a job for about a month at a Jewish sushi bar. Two of my friends came and visited me at work and I gave them free food. It turns out the boss was there; the guy who owned the whole place watched me give free food to my two friends. He came up to me and said, "Let me see the credit card receipt," because I pretended to run it in case anybody was watching and I didn't. I was like "There is none," and he goes, "You're fired." That was the only job I had. I didn't try to get another job. I was still running out of money and I ended up living on oatmeal for a couple of months until my sister visited and bought me groceries. It was horrible.

It must have been in July when the lease was ending. I sold my bed. It was an expensive bed. I bought it when I had financial aid. One of my friends was nice enough to buy it because they needed a new bed and I gave it to her for $500, where she would have to buy a new bed for $1,000. Everyone knows used beds only sell for $200 or $300. She was nice and she gave me $500. I remember the first thing I went and bought was at Jack In the Box and it was so good. I ended up moving back to Northern California. I ended up moving in with my sister. My sister got me a job working at a grocery store. We were both butchers' assistants. People tend to like me right off the bat. They get this gut feeling about me. Even when they don't like other people, they tend to like me. I have to say I like it, but the manager of the grocery store that we worked at, she hated everybody. She met me and she goes, "I want to give you a job."

They had this work event. I don't remember if I worked there at the time or if it was before I started working there, but we ended up going to an A's game and tailgating. I wasn't 21 yet. They were feeding me booze and I was drinking it hard. I hadn't eaten anything all day, let alone water. We were doing the beer bongs. There was this thing called votang. It was vodka, Tang, and vanilla. It tastes exactly like Tang, but it is strong and full of alcohol. I ended up not only peeing my pants on the way to a Porta Potty, because I couldn't hold it; I'm completely drunk. I can't even walk straight. I'm trying to get to the Porta Potty and I can't. Logically, I decided to sit down and pee myself. When I'm sitting there peeing, the dry cement around me, they can see that I'm peeing myself. The assistant store manager walks by. "Are you okay?" he asks. I'm like "Just fine. I'm peeing myself. Can you go over there quickly?" After that happened, I drank some more. I don't remember this part too well because I was blacked out.

We ended up going into the stadium. The game had started, so we were trying to get in. Everybody had to go to the bathroom. When I got to the bathroom, I passed out on the toilet and slipped onto the floor with my pants down. The store manager was in the next stall. I wore glasses and she ended up having to grab my glasses because they called an ambulance and all that stuff. I couldn't see for two days because she had my glasses from saving me from my pants down, passing out on the toilet, which should have been mortifying. It should have been like a wakeup call. Maybe don't drink so much. Your boss, the person who is nice enough to give you a job, saw you blacked out on a toilet with your pants down. You had to go to the hospital for it. That was not anywhere near my end. I did end up going to the hospital. The nurse was not nice and I remember that. I remember him not being nice. He was like "I'm a dad. You're going to pee in this little bin thing." I was like "Okay, I'll pee in it. You don't have to yell at me. I'm trying to sleep here." I went to the hospital that time; it definitely was not great. That was when I was 20.

I lived with my sister. We ended up moving in with her and her fiancé. I turned 21. Nothing too major happened. That was probably the healthiest I've ever been with alcohol. It was directly after I turned 21. I had a twenty-first birthday party. I flirted with some guys. I probably got a little bit too drunk, but it was fine. We ended up moving out to Antioch because he had a house there. There was nothing too horrible. There was one time that we ended up going with a couple of our friends to San Francisco. On the way back, I had a bit too much and I ended up throwing up on myself in the car. It was nothing spectacular, just regular drunk escapades with your sister, your friends, and whatnot. I was more concerned about dating, dieting, and all that stuff. We got a new cat. Life was good at that point. I also decided that I wanted more. I decided let's give college another college try. I applied to SFSU and I got in. I was accepted and I was stoked. I was like "This is going to be my fresh start. This is going to be awesome." I don't even remember what I thought I wanted to be, but I was going to do a business degree or something. I moved from Antioch to San Francisco and that's where everything goes haywire.

I still drink to feel normal. It works for a time, plus everyone loves me being the center of attention, the life of the party, and stuff like that. It's the only other time I've ever had a roommate besides while in recovery, an actual roommate, not a housemate. She was gone the whole time, but I also had other housemates. One of the other housemates was not mentally stable. He was getting in a fight with his girlfriend because she went drinking with me. We didn't get too drunk that time, but he was very controlling. He was pissed. We heard him hit her. We went to the bedroom. Turns out he had taken a mug and smashed it over her head. I'm not familiar with this. I've never been surrounded by violence or drugs, just weirdness. We were like "You can't do that. You've got to stop." He pushes me into the bathroom and he gets really close to my face. He's like "I'm going to kill you." He's right there and I am not going to lie. I'm pretty brave, but that scared me. I don't know when I've ever been so scared. The second he left, I took my stuff and had somebody drive me back to my sister's place because there was no way I was still going to live there. I was so terrified.

My parents allowed me to move back into their place because they wanted me to be able to keep going to school. I was trying to go to class. I wasn't going all the time, but I was making an effort. They said I can move in with them as long as I still went to class and I was trying to get a job. I got a job at Nordstrom. At Nordstrom, I found one of my drinking pals and one of the pals who took me to the darkest depths of drinking that I ever went to. We'll call her N. She and I were trouble together. She usually worked a mid shift and I would close. The problem with that is we were drinking at work. When one of you leaves in the middle of the day and the other one stays until midnight, I have about five hours when I'm alone still drunk and still drinking. She and I would get hammered off of Seagram's Seven. It was cheap and it did the trick.

We worked in a huge mall in San Francisco. We'd find one of the bathrooms downstairs. We'd lock ourselves in the stall. We'd drink in about 10 minutes, back and forth. That seems like it would be fun, but once you started, you can't stop. We'd be taking 10-minute breaks to go smoke a cigarette. To go get shots, to go get another bottle. It was bad. She would leave and she would go home. Now I'm alone and I'm drunk. I want more. I want to get drunker. There were days I don't even know how I got home, honestly. I would come to work almost all the time, praying that I did everything I needed to do not to get fired. Usually, I was proud of myself because even drunk me knew how to get the job done. That's what I always said, "Drunk me knows how to get the job done." I would be drinking by myself a lot. I would go across the street to the liquor store and hang out there with the guy who ran the liquor store for two hours doing nothing, just drinking and smoking cigarettes. I wasn't a smoker, mind you. Nobody in my family I grew up with smokes. I wasn't a smoker, but I liked to smoke, when I drink. If you're drunk all the time, now you're a smoker. I would be smoking and drinking. I never liked how the smoking made me feel, but I did love how the drinking made me feel. At the beginning, when I would smoke and when I drank, it gave me that next level of drunk. You'd be buzzed, then you'd smoke and you'd feel next-level drunk.

Toward the end of my drinking, smoking put me in a blackout. Smoking is horrible. I've never looked up why it does that, but it is terrifying what smoking does to you when you drink. I was a chimney. I did a job where we didn't have to be closely managed. I would stand far away from my manager when they would show up. At that time, I considered myself a functional drinker at work. In my mind, I wasn't even an alcoholic at that point. I was the party girl. I was like "You can always count on Michelle for a good time." I was that girl. I will always go out with you for a drink. I don't say no to drugs. I never got into hard drugs but cocaine. I will do a line with you in the bathroom, "Let's do it." I'm the party girl. I'm the loud girl. I'm the funny girl. I wanted to be it all. I wanted to be everybody's "it" girl.

Almost every night after work, we went to the Castro. There was this little hole-in-the-wall dive bar that we'd go to. They had $2 beers. For $5, you could get a shot and a beer. They had food. I was there every day. I bring people all the time. I was getting free drinks. They knew me there. I didn't have to flash my ID or nothing. I was well-known and I liked it. There were cracks in the façade. There were definitely too many times where I couldn't even get out of bed because I was too hung over. Toward the end, I started drinking a lot by myself and it never went well. I always wanted to be the girl who wears black, who wears leather, and who doesn't take any rubbish because I was always halfway there. I'm pretty self-sufficient. I have great boundaries. I don't need other people. That's how I was raised.

I've seen my mom create boundaries my entire life; even if they didn't make sense, they were there and she would enforce them. That rubbed off on me. I was halfway there, but I wanted the other half. I want to be so cool that everybody wanted to be me and wanted to hang out with me. I thought it was cool to go to a bar and drink by myself.

The image in my head looked great. It's not. I would get so drunk that I would lose bags of stuff. When I say bags of stuff, I'm talking iPads, iPhones, and rent money. I've lost entire months of rent because I was walking on the train tracks and it's gone. I must have tripped and it fell. My drunk self didn't see it and I kept walking home.

There have been times where I took a taxi home. On the way out of the taxi, I tripped and everything scattered on the sidewalk. Instead of picking it all up, I passed out on the sidewalk for about two hours. I woke up, got everything, put it in my bag, and went upstairs. I had been arrested one time for public intoxication, which I still believe is BS because I was sitting outside waiting for this guy. I wasn't being loud or anything. I was sitting there drinking some sake. There was this Japanese guy and he was teaching me a couple of Japanese words, "You're drunk; you're friendly." This other guy walks by and I offered him some sake and he goes, "No." Turns out that guy who walked by was the apartment manager and he called the police. I didn't get arrested. They put me in the drunk tank though.

That time I lost my glasses and I couldn't see for two weeks because I didn't have any glasses. I am the queen of losing stuff when I get drunk. I can't tell you how many iPhones I've lost because I've fallen asleep on public transportation and somebody took it. I was drunk in a cab and I left it. I was drunk in a bar and I lost it. The excuses, they go on. I figured this out, because I had to go back to my apartment and pack up. I was reading my diary. I was wondering why I was missing some games from my Game

Boy. Turns out I got drunk one night and I lost the games. It makes me wonder what else have I forgotten along the way? One thing I've always prided myself on is having a great memory. Alcohol strips that from me so badly. It's like you barely remember your own name. What happened yesterday? I don't know. I have no idea. Long-term, short-term, it doesn't matter. When I read that, my mind was blown because I'd been looking for those Game Boy games for a while. I was like "Where could they have gone?" I ended up happenstance reading my old diary. There is an explanation where these games went. I lost them when I was drunk. When I saw it, I was like "That checks out." I lost everything. I've lost jewelry, money, phones, dignity, and everything is gone.

There are two times that stick out to me. I would always meet people when I used to drink. Because I drank alone, I'd find somebody else who was drunk and then take them with me. It didn't make any sense. They're not real friends. I met this one girl. We were drinking. That's the only way I can explain it. She and I went to a liquor store and got some alcohol. There were these two other girls behind us in line. They had some alcohol with them and they're like "Do you want some of ours?" She and I were both, "Yes, absolutely." The last thing I remember was taking a drink of their alcohol. Turns out they put something in the alcohol. I wouldn't even call it a blackout because it wasn't self-induced; they put drugs in our alcohol. I woke up and I had vomit all over me. All of my stuff was taken. I was looking around. I'm in the same little cubby thing as this homeless guy. I don't know where I am. I was like "What is happening?"

I look at the guy and I'm like "Why am I here?" He goes, "Those two girls jumped you." I was like "I'm sorry, what?" He goes, "Those two girls, they jumped you. They took everything. They searched all your pockets. Everything's gone." The homeless guy gave me his blanket. He felt so bad for me. My phone, my money, all of it was gone. The worst part was I had been losing so many phones that my mom had given me her backup until I could get a new phone. They stole my mom's backup phone and I had to tell her, "I lost another phone," and I couldn't.

I don't even remember to this day if I was honest about how I lost it, if I told her I was drunk or I came up with some story. The stories got so creative because I couldn't be honest with anyone. I couldn't be honest with how drunk I was getting all the time. This wasn't even the worst of my drinking at all. I was so tired from work, I fell asleep at the back of the bus. Some guy took it and he ran off. I chased him and I filed a police report. I was coming up with all these stories and it's hard to keep up with them. Before I was trying to cover up the drinking, I was an honest person. People come to me because they appreciate my honesty and my forwardness. You know you're going to get God's honest truth from me. You know you're going to get 100 percent. I don't BS. You want the truth, you come to me. At this point, it was hard to keep track of all my lies. I felt bad because I'm lying to the people who I care about the most. It occurred to me that if I lied to these people, then I don't care about them.

I would tell N the things I would do and she and I would laugh about it. We'd go get even drunker. I wasn't lying to her because to her it's another drunken story. I got jumped, which sucked. It still didn't hit home for me. Then this one time I know I was drinking at work. And I blacked out. The next thing I know, I'm coming to in a car. I don't know the guy who's driving it. I freak out. I'm like "Let me out of your car. I don't know you. Please let me out." I get out of the car. When the door closed, I realized that I left my entire purse in there. There is an iPad in there. There's money in there. There's everything in there. Fortunately, I had my phone and I had my keys on me. I didn't lose those. Once I got out, I was like "I know where I am." To get to my apartment, you have to go over to this street. It looks like a freeway but it's a street. You walk over to it. You're on the other side. There's my apartment. It's perfect. I know where I am. I'm going to start walking. I start walking over the little hill thing.

About 25 minutes later, I realized I'm walking barefoot on the freeway. This was not where I thought it was. I had entered the freeway and I'm now walking in the middle of the freeway. I don't know where I am. Cars are honking as they pass me. I turn and then there's this car. They pull over and there are these two guys in there. They're like "What are you doing? You're in the middle of the freeway." I was like "I am." They're like "Get in our car. We'll give you a ride home." I'm in the middle of the freeway. I don't have a choice. I'm still drunk. I'm like "I'll get in the car." These guys drive around downtown. The one guy gets dropped off and then the other guy goes and parks and pulls out a meth pipe. He starts smoking meth in the car. Mind you, I don't smoke meth. I don't do meth. I'm like "What is happening?" Then he goes, "You're going to light it for me now." He gave me the lighter and he made me light his meth pipe. He goes, "If you light my meth pipe, we can go home now." I was like "What is happening?"

I'm so far from home that I can't get out and get lost. I don't have any money on me. I was like "Fine." I'm in the backseat. He's in the front seat. Finally, he stopped smoking meth. We're driving around and I'm still drunk. I end up passing out. When I wake up, he's masturbating in the front seat. I was like "What are you doing? Are you serious right now?" He goes, "Yes, when you bent over I saw your panties." I was like "I want to go home. You made me light your meth pipe. Now you're jerking off in the front seat." He goes, "Would you believe if I told you I haven't done this in several years?" I was like "No," and then I look around and I'm like "I know where I am." I'm still drunk, though. Instead of being like "I'm out," I was like "You either drive me home right now or I'm getting out and walking." I don't know why that's an ultimatum for him, but he ended up driving me to my house and dropping me off. I never saw that guy again. That was a crazy thing. I go to bed and I wake up. I end up not telling my sister about this for a long time, but I tell N. We laugh about it because we laugh at all of these stories because they're ridiculous.

There was one time that she got too drunk and I was trying to get her home. She punched me straight in the face and I got a black eye. That was not fun. We had tons of stories like that where either she's overly intoxicated or I am. Mine go to the extreme. I was walking on the freeway.

That still blows my mind. There was a time when I first moved to San Francisco, and my sister had broken up with her fiancé. She ended up moving in with me, which I thought was going to make me the happiest person. I love my sister. She's my favorite person. She's funny and she's smart. All I ever wanted to do was spend time with her, but the drinking got in the way. At a certain point, I was like "You've got to get out. Go find your own place." I got tired of her always caring about me. It gets in the way of you doing what you want to do. When people care, you've got to make excuses. It was either create space between us or lie to her. I didn't want to lie to her. I'm tired of lying to the people who I love and who love me too. I told her, "I don't want to text you good night anymore. If I don't text good night, then you're worried about me."

Nowadays, that would never be a problem. If she wanted to text good night every night, we shouldn't have to be required to say it. I didn't want it to be a rule then because if I blacked out and didn't say it, I didn't want her to worry. The amount of time that I showed up drunk and covered in vomit on her door was so much, It didn't equate. Either I want space, or I need her. I kept doing it, and I feel so bad about the amount of stuff that I put her through, it was crazy. She definitely didn't deserve it, and she didn't know how to handle it. She's a person who gets her feeling hurt easily and she is an anxious person and to be like "I'm not going to tell you where I am anymore, that I'm safe or that I'm alive. Deal with it." That's BS. I wanted freedom. I wanted to do whatever I wanted to do and I didn't want anyone to tell me any different. I needed to feel normal and I was going to do whatever I needed to do that. I wanted to feel I was on top of the world and screw anybody who got in the way. She was always cautious. I wanted to try cocaine and I wanted to be out partying. She wanted to be a little bit safer and I was like "God, I need freedom."

I ended up getting fired from Nordstrom. We were so shocked. I spent a few months finding another job. I ended up getting a restaurant job. I was hired as a host. About a month later, they made me a manager. That's quite a big leap. They liked how I did my business, I got it done. The restaurant business is full of alcohol and it is full of drugs. It is full of people who behave badly. It's full of sex, booze, parties, and all the wrong things. That's when everything started to rev up a little bit. Looking back now, I can see it. Now, having gone through treatment and all that stuff, you can see glaring signals and all of the signs. But I was blind to it. When I went from host to manager, it played with my whole wanting-to-be-accepted thing. All these servers and bartenders don't want the girl who is a host telling them what to do. I desperately wanted friends. I wanted to be liked. I wanted everyone to know how great I was. Instead of being a good manager, I was a good friend. I drank with them. I did drugs with them. I went out with them. I didn't ever get them in trouble for all the things that I should have. As a manager, they got themselves in trouble, but being on time, not doing the correct thing, all of that stuff. I never did anything. I let them do whatever the hell they wanted. I did the manager stuff. I count the money, did all the paperwork, and stuff like that. I wanted to be friends with all of them so bad that I never followed up.

We were all getting super-drunk at work. We used to have a code word for cocaine. Whenever anybody would go get some coke, we'd say, "Do you want some steak tacos?" That meant "I have coke. Would you like some?" Me and another manager, he was way heavier into the drinking than I was at that time. He couldn't even go a day or an hour without drinking on the job or he'd start shaking. He would do coke all the time. I used to do coke with N. I tried it first with her and I loved that. I thought it was great, but I started to use it too much, so I stopped. I was like "I'm good." I would hate to become a cokehead. God forbid I have a problem. God forbid I end up like my biological parents. I end up stopping all that. I don't want to be that person, but drinking never occurred to me like "Maybe I should slow down a little bit," because it was a part of my identity. It was a part of who I was. It was part of how I define myself. I could drink anyone under the table. I'll drink anytime, anywhere; it doesn't matter. I'm the fun girl. That was who I was. If I didn't have that, what did I have?

When I started working at the restaurant, my other manager, he would get an eight ball and we would do it all sitting in his car. That will mess with you. You go back into work. You want a shot. You want a cigarette. I'm outside chain-smoking because my mouth is numb, but it feels great. I want to smoke. I want another shot. An hour would have gone by, and I'm like "What is going on?" All of a sudden, we're closed. I'm drinking stuff from behind the bar to stay drunk. It's 2:00 a.m. I can't buy alcohol anywhere. I'll drink the stuff at work. I was not a good employee by any means. I couldn't be because I was desperate to fit in. I would hang out with the kitchen guys. I would hang out with the servers.

It's taken a long time for me to realize that none of them were my friends, not even a little bit—not in that they didn't care about me, they cared about me at that moment, but not long-term, not in the way that friendship does. It was more they wanted something to talk about. I was the next best thing to talk about. Believe me, I gave them the stuff to talk about. That's not on them; that's definitely on me. After things happen, because of Facebook and Instagram, you always want to keep in touch and see how they're doing. I kept these people around me for too long when all I have associated with them are these bad memories of being too drunk, doing the wrong thing and doing too much coke. The restaurant industry is hard and fast. It'll chew you up. It'll spit you out. You've got to be careful. I wanted to be chewed up and spit out. I wanted to go do the drinking scene. I want to do the drugs. I wanted to do all of it.

At a certain point, I was like "Enough is enough. I don't like who I am as a person. I've got to start doing better." I got a better restaurant job, but I told myself, "I'm going to stop smoking," because where I was going to work, if you wanted to smoke, it would take you 15 minutes to get outside to smoke. I was like "This is a great opportunity. I'll stop smoking. I'm going to do all the right things at work, like no shady stuff, no drinking at work, no drinking their alcohol, none of that." I was going to start making more money, being

343

a better friend, being a better sister. It all started out great.

I'll rewind a little bit. I ended up dating a guy who worked for me at the restaurant. He and I, as all my stories start, were drinking together. I believe our story started with me throwing up on him. The best of love stories start that way. At the time that he and I started hooking up, I lived with one of my other managers. She was not a very good person, but I didn't realize that at the time. I was a huge fan of her. I thought she was great. I thought she was the coolest. It was in my best interest to be around her. The reason I ended up becoming a manager was that I hung out with her and I told her, "If you guys need help, let me know. I'd be happy to be a manager for you guys." I ended up getting it because she suggested me to one of the regional managers and they're like "Let's interview her," and they liked me. I was like "I'll be around her and I'll do whatever she wants. I'll be a great friend and all that stuff." It turns out everything was about her.

My nephew ended up dying in 2014. I saw that as a personal thing. I wanted to handle it personally. I wasn't close to him, but that was still shocking for me. She went and told everybody. I couldn't believe that she would do that. She ended up telling my regional manager, who pulled me aside to talk about it, which I thought was incredibly inappropriate because I was like "I didn't tell you this. She told you this. I don't need you talking to me about this in any way, shape, or form." That's the person she was. She would say stuff to get attention. I thought I was being slick by dating the guy from work. Employees are not supposed to date. I would have him come over to my house all the time. She would go walk the dogs and smoke. I'd sneak him in and we'd be in the other room. He would Spider-Man his way out of the building on the outside, on the ladders. It was our little secret. Turns out it wasn't that much of a secret. Everybody knew. Everybody talks about everything. I found out a couple of years later that he was telling everybody.

He and I ended up moving in together. We lived in an SRO, single room occupancy. You share a bathroom with a bunch of people on your same floor but you have your own room. He and I lived there together. We were not healthy for each other. We did not eat well. We did none of the right things. We were together out of convenience. I'd never had a real boyfriend before and I wanted to see what it was like. It's not great. We tried to make it work. There were some big things that were never going to work. He was one of the first people to tell me to my face, "You need to stop drinking. You have a problem." I did not want to hear that. I would tell him that I feel I have a lot of issues and I want to go get help like therapy. He told me, "That's stupid and you shouldn't do that." I had a cabbie pull me aside one time and be like "You shouldn't be with this guy. A guy who tells you not to take care of your mental health probably isn't the guy for you." He comes back all like "What did you say to my girl?" and he was trying to fight him. I was like "This is so embarrassing."

Another big thing was he wanted to own a gun and I said, "I don't feel comfortable living in a house that has a gun in it," and he brought home a gun. I said, "What is this? You need to respect my wishes because I do not feel comfortable." He told me that he brought it to his friend's house. That it was all good and it was gone. I trusted him. Weirdly enough, I don't have trust issues. I take people at face value because I assume you're telling the truth. I certainly don't have relationship issues. I wouldn't be with you if I didn't think that you were 100 percent with me. I'm not going to go through your phone. He always wanted to go through my phone, which is ridiculous. There was nothing wrong with him doing it, because he wasn't going to find anything, but I knew that was an unhealthy boundary. He shouldn't be doing that. We'd fight a lot about stuff like that because it's like "Stop wanting to go through my phone, stop making me defend myself, stop making it look like I'm guilty, because I don't want you to go through my things." He recorded me one time when he went to work. He had an iPad and he put it on record the whole time to see if I was cheating, which I wasn't. I should have broken up with him when I found that out. We weren't a match. We were trying to make it work so hard and it wasn't.

I ended up starting my new job at a new restaurant and I was trying to be better. I was working 13-hour days five days a week. Coming home, I was tired. I'm coming home at 5:00 in the morning, tired and stressed. He would want me to make him dinner, a sandwich or something. He only worked five hours a day and I'm like "You want me to make something for you?" I always had to tell him where I was. That's when his and my relationship started to not work so much. He ended up moving out of the SRO. The day that he moved out, he moved all of his stuff out. He walks back in.

I'm crying because I know it should happen, but I'm still sad. He looks at me dead in the eye. He reaches on top of our closet, which I couldn't reach the top of because I'm short. He pulls down the gun. He looks me dead in the eye and then walks out the door.

I couldn't believe that this whole time instead of being honest with me and instead of getting rid of the gun, he put it on top, where he knew I couldn't reach it. He knew that the whole time and yet he would call me a liar and he would always be questioning me and doing stuff when in actuality he's the one doing shady stuff. I found out when we were first together he'd slept with somebody else. It was crazy, but he was the first person to tell me I got to get my drinking together. I would wake up and he would be like "Do you remember?" and I'd wake up in a great mood. I'm like "Give me a kiss," and he's like "You don't remember last night, do you?" I'm like "No." We would get in fights in public. I would tell him he doesn't care about me.

He always hated that I told him that I don't care if I'm going to die soon, die young because we're all going to die sometime and I never expected to live that long. It's true. I never expected to live that long. I don't know why, but I had this sneaking suspicion that I'm going to die young, with no backup evidence whatsoever. It's a crazy thought. I told him that once and it pissed him off. I wouldn't want to stick around and be with him forever. Apparently, when I got drunk, I would taunt him about that. I'm sure he never told me the full story, because I can't remember, but I know how he manipulates the truth. I'm still waking up from a blackout and I have no idea. It was not good. The number of times we were in public and I'm screaming at him or he's fighting with me over nothing.

When I first started at the new restaurant, I did well. I did stop drinking for a while. Even though he wanted me to quit drinking, he would tell me that I wasn't that fun because I didn't want to go out drinking because I was tired. It was weird and backward, so we ended up breaking up. After we broke up, I ended up moving in with one of my coworkers because he worked in the kitchen. He was a kitchen manager and I was the front house manager. We go through the same stuff, as we tend to have the same schedule. It was perfect. We could commute to work. He and I would drink together after work sometimes. At first, it wasn't that bad, but then life catches up with you in weird sorts of ways. By this point, I'm 27, 28. I feel a lot more comfortable with myself. I'm coming to terms with the fact that I am weird and that's okay. I still do things a lot of times to feel like I have friends or to feel popular. Drinking for me is an absolute crutch. My anger as well, I wouldn't say anger management issues, but I have a short temper and I use it as a weapon. I use it to keep people at bay, because if you're mad at them, it keeps them on their toes. I know how to use it to manipulate people, I always have and I've always used it that way.

I don't feel proud of myself at this point as a person because I tried to go back to school and I had failed. I have a ton of student debt. If I'm being honest with everyone; I have $43,000 in student loans that I have to pay back. What that $43,000 in student loans bought me is an addiction to alcohol. It bought me coke and bought me a ton of alcohol for a long period of time. I realized that I don't like being a restaurant manager. I start to hate myself because I realize I don't have a chance at another career unless I stick to this. This is one of the only careers I can have without a degree and go far and make a ton of money. Money for me was a driving factor for a long time because my biological parents are poor, but my aunt and uncle, who adopted me, my mom and dad, are well-off. I want to be like them. I want to make a lot of money.

In my head, I'm correlating the two. You guys are not successful and in my head you guys are losers. You never tried to do anything with yourself. On the other hand, we have people here who have a great work ethic. They have a lot of money. They seem happy to me. They've been together forever. That's what I want. I correlate being a winner and being successful with money. You can't have one without the other. You cannot be successful if you do not have money. The idea of being successful without money was hard to wrap my head around

I was making myself do this and I was breaking my back for this company. I was working 13-hour days. I was there until 5:00 in the morning. I was doing all the hard work. I was doing the backbreaking work. We'd be scrubbing dishes, labeling stuff, covering stuff, and cleaning stuff until 5:00 in the morning, only to wake up to a text at 7:00 a.m. that said, "You left two dirty dishes." "With how hard I worked, that's all you have to say to me?" It was supposed to be a motivational technique. Tell them they're not good enough, they'll work harder and it worked. I was there. I was doing it. I kept doing it. I was making myself miserable doing this because I couldn't imagine a life outside of this. What am I going to do, a Customer Service job forever? That's what I'm going to do forever, the thing that I hate. This is my only chance to move up to corporate because I knew I couldn't do college. I don't have it in me. It's not going to happen.

To deal with the stress, my roommate and I were enablers. We both deal with the same stress. We're like "We'll get drunk together," but the problem is he would drink and go to bed. I would drink and drink until there's no more to drink. If I blacked out between now and the end of the bottle, I'd wake up and finish the rest of the bottle. I'm not going to work with this much Jameson left. That's going to be gone. It got to the point where he's going to work hungover and I'm going to work still drunk because I'm going to find the rest of the bottle. I'm going to finish it before we get in the cab to get to work. The quality of my work went down.

Toward the end, I was almost having an identity crisis because I knew I didn't want to do this. I knew this would make me miserable for the rest of my life, but I knew to quit would make me miserable. I'm stuck between this rock and a hard place. I'm getting drunk all the time. I would hide shots in my boobs because they are big enough. I can walk in and I'd go to the bathroom, take the shots, and get back to work. I'm showing up drunk and I'm staying drunk. It's getting to the point where I drink to forget what I did and then

I'll do something else stupid, so I'll drink to forget that. It's an ongoing thing.

Toward the end, I don't respect who I was as a manager. The team members deserve better than what I was giving them. I couldn't give them better. I had to keep not feeling stuff. If I felt anything, I'd feel embarrassed and tons of regret. There's no way. I'm that type of person where I will get to a decision and it's happening now. I can't wait to do it. I can't think it through. Once I've made up my mind, that's it. It's final. I showed up. I took everything out of my box and threw it in a bag. I did inventory for them. I did the right thing. I'm not going to screw them over that bad. I threw all my stuff in the bag and I left. Somebody texted me like "Why is your box empty?" I was like "I quit," and then my dad called me and he goes, "You probably shouldn't quit right off the bat. You should probably give them two weeks' notice." I was like "Okay." I was sick and they wouldn't let me stay home and take care of myself. I had strep throat and they wouldn't let me stay home and take care of myself. They're like "We'll see you tomorrow." I have strep throat. What part of "Can I take care of myself?" Do you not understand? I texted him and I was like "I still don't feel well and this is my two-week notice."

I thought quitting was going to be the thing that would save me. Turns out when you quit the job that you thought was the only career you could ever have without a degree, you feel like a huge loser, especially when your next job is a cashier position. I was a manager of a $21-million restaurant and I'm ringing you up for $7.51. I did not feel good. I would try to control my drinking. At this point, I still haven't come to terms at all with the fact that I have a drinking problem in any way, shape, or form. I know I probably drink more than normal people, and I knew that I drink for the wrong reasons. I wasn't like "This is problematic." I still thought I can stop whenever I want. I've got control over this. I would try to drink less. It would work for a little bit, but then there would come these binges. I would start drinking and I wouldn't be able to stop. I would show up to work drunk, which makes no sense. I don't know why I can come to work drunk, they're going to know. I'm doing my best, but instead, I never got fired. I tried to stay one step ahead of the curve. I'd quit. I would tell them, "This isn't the job for me." I'd quit before they could fire me. I was like "You're not going to fire me. I'm too smart for that." I ended up quitting three jobs. I found this great job. It was easy. It paid well. It gave me sick leave.

Around this time, I thought I might have a problem because I ended up Face-Timing my parents and being like "I have a problem." They suggested AA and I was like "Okay." I went to one meeting. It was not for me. I was like "This is weird. This is super- religious." It was demeaning. It was held inside a church and I was like "I don't think so." Instead, I did the SMART program or at least I started to. I didn't follow up at all. I was like "I'm going to quit drinking for a year. That's what I'm going to do. I'm going to quit drinking for a year; that way, I can get back in control of my life." I wasn't super far off the mark with this one. I knew that if I could start to fix things in my life and be proud of myself, I could do better. The problem is I became a dry drunk. I wasn't working on any of the problems. The only thing that I had to be proud of was the fact that I wasn't drinking. I stopped drinking for a few months. I felt more clearheaded. My memory was starting to come back, that memory that I'm proud of. I'm pretty sarcastic, but I'm pretty whip-smart too. I can come back with a response like that. I lost that when I was drinking because I had trouble thinking of words a lot. I was like "Never mind," and I couldn't think of it. It's not funny when all you got is "Never mind."

It was coming back to me. I was feeling good. I start to feel left out, because all my friends were drinking. I thought I have a couple months under my belt. I'll drink a little bit. I'll drink for this week and then I'll go back to it and I'll finish the year. I went back for that week and that was the worst week of my entire life. I have never been so drunk or blacked out for so long. I hid bottles. The problem also with living in San Francisco is they deliver alcohol to your front door. I didn't know how to drive. When I was a kid, one of the punishments that my parents had for me was "We're not going to teach you to drive anymore," so I never learned to drive, even though it's something that I've always wanted. When you're too busy drinking and feeling sorry for yourself, you don't tend to go out there and accomplish things in life. I never got my license. I don't have any DUIs. I've never been arrested. I got put in the drunk tank at one time, but I don't have any charges. I don't have drunk in public. I don't have any of that. My name's not in the system for any reason, and mostly that's because I could order and I could say, "Bring it to my couch." I could order endlessly and I wouldn't have to go anywhere. I would get it delivered to my front door. I would order and order.

When you're ordering, you're ordering a handle and you're like "I can't handle a handle. I'm going to die if I drink a handle." Instead, I would get the little 250 milliliters and I would hide one. I'd drink this one, and then once that one was done, I'd wake up. I'd find the next one and I'd start drinking that one until I blacked out. I'd wake up and I'd do it all over again. I ended up going into one of the longest blackouts and I drank until I couldn't physically drink anymore. I stood up. and that was the moment in my life, the exact moment that I knew that I had to get help. I stood up and I looked around me. I'd quit my job, yet again because I was too drunk to go in. I was honest with her too. I texted her and I said, "I can't come in because I'm too drunk. I apologize," and I avoided talking to her ever again. I didn't have rent for the next month because I spent every penny of it on booze. You're paying double when you're getting stuff delivered because of the delivery fee. The amount of money I wasted and then the food for when you're hungover, it's horrible and the money for the Uber to go get it.

I stood up, looked around me. This was March of 2018. I hated everything that I saw. I saw myself. I saw everything that I had worked for slipping through my fingers. I didn't have any money. I couldn't pay rent. I feel a sense of responsibility to my roommate. He's one of my best friends. We're on the lease together. I can't screw him over like that and get us kicked out. I had my bank account closed because I couldn't pay it. I wasn't able to hang out with my parents or my sister because I was ashamed of myself and everything I was going through. I didn't have a job. I couldn't be around my friends. I didn't feel I could be my true self around my friends because I'm continually getting drunk. I don't have anything to offer in the relationship because all I am is a drunk. I hated it. I was like "Maybe I need someone else to help me." I started to look for rehabs. I didn't want to do outpatient. I knew that I needed to do something where I moved in, not only because I needed the intensive care, but also the attention and the constant supervision.

I wanted to leave San Francisco. I needed to leave San Francisco. I couldn't stay there and be ashamed of myself. In order to get better, I knew I had to be at a place where I didn't feel judged. Nobody knew what I'd done, what I had been through or any of that stuff. I could start clean. That was important to me. I don't know why I chose Santa Cruz. I didn't choose any other city outside of Santa Cruz. I called places in San Francisco and in Santa Cruz. Here's what they don't tell you about getting help. It is hard. You can ask a thousand times for help and receive a thousand "No's." That to me was frustrating. I'm calling and they're saying, "We'll give you a call back," because I didn't have insurance. I barely have any money. I have a little bit left in this medical account that I had at the restaurant. It was about to expire soon, so I was like "I've got to get this going." I was getting so frustrated because every single place was a "no". The only yes I got was from New Life Treatment Center in Santa Cruz. I went to go sell some of my stuff to pay for the transportation to get there. I figured if I get into a place in

Santa Cruz I'm going to need a bus ticket. I don't drive. I'm certain at this point not going to burden anybody who I know with getting me there because I know I have to do this myself. I have to get myself there and do this myself so I can show people I want this and I am worthwhile.

No one was still getting back to me. It's super-frustrating. I still hadn't heard back. Everyone had said no. I sold my stuff. I was at McDonald's. I'm sitting there. I've never been homeless. I've been far from homeless. My parents were pretty well off. I've been fortunate in my life to never be anywhere near that. My low, my down and out, my lowest point looks different from other people's because of the quality of life I've been very fortunate to have. I knew I was at my lowest point when I thought I was going to be homeless. That to me was unacceptable. That was embarrassing to me like how am I going to lie to my parents about this one? How could I possibly lie to them? What's the lie going to be? I had a plan too. I was going to join a gym and I was going to keep my stuff there because you can shower. You can sleep there, you can work out, and you can shower and go find a job, until you can get money for an apartment. I had a plan because I couldn't fathom the idea of being an actual homeless person. I don't know if my family would have let me do that, but I wasn't about to test it. I was ashamed of myself at that point. I couldn't imagine that anybody else liked me. I thought I didn't like myself because no one else liked me. I thought no one liked me because I didn't like myself. It was the total opposite.

I had pushed everything to the absolute limits that I could without hating myself. Honestly at this point, I wanted things to end. I wanted to die, so I wouldn't have to experience this anymore, so this would end. I wanted it to end already. It was a miserable existence, drinking all the time. When I first started drinking, I thought it was awesome. You're drunk and all this stuff. Living in a constant stupor is horrible. It's not a quality of life that I wish on anybody. A self-induced stupor is horrible. You know that you're doing this to yourself and they make it seem so easy, "Just pull yourself up. Pull yourself out of it." There are so many issues behind it and why I'm here. I have to work on these issues first. Being a dry drunk doesn't work. You got to work on the issues behind it. You are your circumstances, your experiences, the people who raised you, your surroundings. All of that plays into who you are and why you are.

The amount of self-hatred I had at the end was insurmountable. I couldn't imagine that anyone loved me still. I thought my parents hated me. I thought my sister hated me. I couldn't see why they would love me because I've been a bad person. I'd been flaky. I'd been a liar. I know they're not stupid. They know I've lied to them. I'm at McDonald's. In my head, I'm like "If I'm going to be homeless, this thing I never thought I'd be, and is horrible, I might as well get drunk, so I don't remember I have to be homeless." I was thinking, I'll hide in my room, so my roommate can't see me. He sees that I'm drinking again and I was like "There's a liquor store up the street. There's a liquor store over there." I'm planning what size bottle I'm going to get because I still wanted money in my pocket when I become homeless for food or whatever.

I'm standing up to throw out my tray and the intake supervisor calls me right when I'm standing up to go get more alcohol. Not before, not after. As I'm making up my mind to go get more alcohol, she calls me. She goes, "We might have space for you." That was the first yes I'd heard. I was like "Are you kidding me?" On top of that, that medical account that I had $733 in. Do you know how much it costs to get into New Life? $700. That for me was such a huge sign that I was doing exactly what I was supposed to do. I've never been drug-tested before. When I went to treatment, I did it on my own terms. I've never had to go to jail or anything like that. I don't know how drug tests work. I'm thinking they can go far back. I was like "I'll make sure not to drink because I don't want to not get in." I ended up taking three different buses, Amtrak, BART, and walking to get there. It takes me five hours to get there, but I did it. I packed my suitcase. I packed all my stuff. I found a roommate for my roomie so that he didn't have to move out. I did all of this. I wanted this so bad because I didn't want to be that person anymore. I knew I've always had potential. I've always seen who I could be. I hadn't met my potential yet. I knew I had to be a different person. I couldn't spend the rest of my life or even the rest of my twenties. I only got a year left, but I can't spend the rest of my twenties wasted and drunk. I couldn't.

I get to New Life Treatment Center in Santa Cruz, California. I excelled there for three reasons: I put myself there, I chose to be there, and I searched for this place. And I was stoked when they said "yes." Only one other place ever called me back. This person called me in June and was like "Do you still need a place?" If I'd still been out there drinking, I would be dead by now. Thank you for your help, but no, I don't still need a place. I stopped drinking in March. I got into New Life in March. I wanted to be there. I live here. I've agreed to these rules. I'm going to do well because I know I agreed to that. I'm going to follow the rules. I don't make my own rules. Otherwise, I would live in my own house. I do well when there's outside supervision and all that stuff. Lastly, because I knew if I didn't do this and I failed or my definition of fail, I would be homeless. That was not an option. That option didn't make sense to me. I don't know how to do it. I couldn't do it. I said, "No" to that option. I went to New Life Treatment Center and it literally changed my life.

The 12-Step program, when I first got there, I definitely thought it was religious. There's still a part of me that thinks it is. I didn't find my higher power, but it was there all along. I knew it was there all day long. I cut off the communication. Drinking, you can't hear your higher power. No ifs ands or buts about it. You're deaf. I always had a higher power. I've always believed in a higher power, so that one was easy for me. I don't believe that I'm the highest thing out there. That's stupid. Look at me. It did seem religious but you know what I knew. I knew if I went in and I rearranged my thinking, if I took what they were telling me and I made it self-applicable, I could make it work for me. Everything they said didn't have to be 100 percent true, but I had to make it work for me, and that's what I did. I took everything that they said and I learned something from it. Even if it wasn't exactly what they were saying, I made it apply to my life and I made it work.

I had six months in October. That time has flown but I have done more in those several months than I have in the many years of my life. I learned to drive and I got my driver's license. I start real estate school next week so I can have a career that I don't need to go get a degree for. I'm a manager again at a restaurant so I can do the job that I know I am capable of doing and can do it well and be successful and do the job that I'm supposed to do. I show up. I'm on time. I'm responsible. I have a purpose. My dad used to talk to me about priorities and how I didn't have mine straight. I didn't know what he meant because I felt like I was always focusing on all the right things. The problem is I wasn't doing all the right things. Even though I think about all these things I should be doing and my focus is always on it because I'm like, "I need to do this," it doesn't mean I was doing it though.

Now, I am doing the right thing. I'm always doing the next best thing. When someone asks me to do something, I say yes and I show up. I show up on time. I offer to help when I can. I do the best that I can every single moment. I've never loved myself as much as I love myself now. That has been a huge part of my recovery. I'm so far from the person who walked in those doors. I'm full of hope. I would be dead without this program. I'm eternally grateful because it's been a complete 180. A huge problem that I used to have before with myself is that I would say I wanted to do something or that I would do something and I would never do it. I couldn't even trust myself because I can never seem to follow through because drinking would always get in the way.

Nowadays, I don't even know how I had time for drinking. My life is full in such an amazing way—it's beautiful. There's never a day that I'm not doing something; I'm doing this, I'm doing meetings, I'm doing work. I'm going on a road trip with my sister, stuff like that. We would say we would do it, but we'd never do it. Now we're doing it. I get to go driving whenever I want. Life is beautiful now. My vision was shaded before; I couldn't see anything clearly. My priorities are in line. I'm grateful. I'm humble. I'm happy. I could not wish for anything more. It's been 29 years to get here, but I know that the journey I took to get here was what it was meant to be. Every step of the way, from my parents being drug addicts, to being molested, to living with my aunt and uncle, who had weird rules, but my best intentions at heart, to failing out of college, all of that led me to this moment here and this amount of happiness. That's what I got.

Thank you so much, Michelle. To our readers, stay sober and be happy.

7. Andrea: Female, 43, A Mother on Meth

I'll be talking to Andrea about her addiction and her recovery from addiction. Andrea is a client at Gault House Sober Living Environment in Santa Cruz. Andrea is 43 years old and from San Francisco's South Bay Silicon Valley area. Andrea has 11 days clean.

Andrea, welcome to the interview.

Thank you.

Andrea, how did your addiction start?

It was basically a party-scene type of thing. It was Thursday night, Friday night, Saturday, Sunday, and when all my friends went to work on Monday, I only did that for a little while. I couldn't go back to work because I would carry my partying into my weekdays and I never stopped. I was different from my friends in that way.

How old were you when you first started your addiction?

I was about 23 years old. I was a young mom at 19 when I had my first baby. I'm married as well. When my first one was one-year-old, we found out I was pregnant with my second. They're only 20 months apart. I had two kids at the age of 21.

Why do you think you used drugs?

I didn't realize that I had addiction problems while I was in it the first go around. I've been in the program for a while. I realized that it had a lot to do with my upbringing. I was raised by my stepdad and my mom in a church that was pretty much a cult. I was unable to have a normal life as the kids did who I went to school with. It had an impact on me as far as my happiness. I was miserable as a child. I had fun sometimes, but looking back now I walked on eggshells. I was not a normal kid. I moved out of the house when I was 17. I was working full-time while the rest of my friends were in college, but I was okay with that because I could not live by my parents' rules anymore. I ended up getting married young and started around 23 when my husband and I got a divorce or at least separated. I started meeting new people and going out. I hit the San Francisco party scene pretty hard and I got to know a lot of people. It was easy to get out there and to party with them. Everything was readily available, so I never had a hard time finding a good time.

It started out with drinking, weed, and coke. It got a little bit more hardcore with the methamphetamines and the GHB, Special K, a lot of Ecstasies. For some reason, the meth was something I could not put down. I gave it several years of my life from about the age of 23 to 32. It was a while and I was a daily user. I got to the point where I couldn't even function without it. I lost many jobs. I'm a very dependable employee when I'm sober, but that stuff got me. I was not able to even hold down a job. I was skinny at the time. I had expired tags on my car. The first thing that happened was a bicycle cop was in the parking lot waiting for me because I had expired tags on my car. He called back up. They searched my car. They found meth in my car and I went to jail for the first time.

That was not a wakeup call. I didn't even show up to court. I could have got a deferment the judge said. Instead, I had to end up hiring a lawyer because I had a warrant out for my arrest and they gave me Prop 36. In Prop 36, I had to go to these meetings. At the time, I'd only snorted meth. I ended up meeting people who are more hardcore who shot it and smoked it. That began my smoking run with methamphetamines and it was a good one. A lot happened during that time. My kids' dad and I were in a custody battle. I thought I was fooling everybody, but the only person I was fooling was me when I'd go into the courtroom looking strung out. The judge was good to me in the fact that he gave me half custody of my girls. We shared physical and legal custody of the girls. I couldn't stop it and I would be late to pick them up. I was not reliable.

It got to the point where they didn't even want to be with me. There was a time where I couldn't pay my bills and the electricity was shut off. I ended up getting an eviction notice and I lost my place. That resulted in me having to give the kids up to my ex-husband and living in a car. I did that for about a year and I did not want help. I wanted to stay in the life where I knew I'd be able to get high every day. I never resorted to selling myself or anything like that. It was an embarrassing situation. I wouldn't even call it humbling because it was ugly. I was hanging out with whoever I knew had it and I had no morals, no dignity, and I'd lost who I was. I ended up going to Turlock into this home and you had to be sober to live there. It was different from Gault House. It was run by some jerks and I was unhappy there. I stuck it out for three months. Even when I got out of there, I still used.

My parents wouldn't take me back in. I didn't have anywhere to go, but I had this one friend who is still in my life now. He was loving enough to take me in. He lived in Modesto at the time. I went ahead and lived with him and his mom and his stepdad. It was humbling for me because I felt low and I still didn't want to stop using. I managed to find it wherever it was that I went. We at one point ended up at his sister's place in Mountain View and I continued to use. If I go back, there was a man in my life or a guy in my life who I was seeing while I was using. I felt funny and I went to the doctor. I was stepping on the scale and I was 85 pounds. This was at the age of 30. It ended up I was pregnant. I didn't know what to do. There's no way that the baby was going to be okay. I had used every day all day for years. I had a decision to make, which was one of the hardest ones in my life. I know a lot of women go through it, but I couldn't go through with the thought of bringing somebody into this world I had hurt already before they were even formed.

I still feel it was the right thing to this day and decided not to go through with having the baby. That is something that haunts me all the time. The reason I go back to this is that I was still using when I was living at his sister's house in Mountain View. He and I were still together off and on. We were off and on for years before that. I've known him for many years. He was not a user. He is a "normie," but he loved me. He would take the bad and the good; whatever I could give, he would take. I was using and thin and a rack of bones again years later. I should know because I already had two kids and they're healthy and they're wonderful. I thought I knew my body. I'm a hypochondriac, so I think something's wrong with me all the time. I don't know why I didn't know, but I was cramping badly. There was no sign of pregnancy at all and this is years later. I went to the restroom and miscarried right at that point. The Fire Department came first. The ambulance came. I had to go to the hospital. All these things were going on that I was doing to myself, self-sabotage because I could not stop using methamphetamines. It was killing me. It was making it so that nothing happy was happening in my life.

For somehow, some way, I cleaned up for about a month and I got a job. I was getting over that trauma. I worked there, and I was clean for a while, but it would be weekends or whenever I could get my hands on something, I'd still use that meth. I basically was working for this company in the Accounts Payable department and I had a company credit card. This is one of the most embarrassing and shameful things I've ever done and I'm still paying for it to this day. I got caught up using the card for personal purchases and ended up getting caught and going to jail. I served some time for that. I knew I needed to be bailed out because I had court on a certain date, a little bit after I was booked. It was to get my youngest daughter back. She did not want to stay with her dad and his girlfriend anymore. I knew I had to get out of jail in order to be able to make it to court and to get her back. She was depending on me. I was able to get bailed out and make that court date. I got her back and that's when I got clean. It was a miracle to me that I was able to get her back that easy, one court date. It was honored and I had nothing but happiness and thankfulness in my heart.

At that point is finally when I got clean from methamphetamines and never used again. It caused me to lose my children. It caused me to lose several jobs. It caused me to lose my place. It caused me to lose myself. It caused me to miscarry and have to give up a baby. It caused me a felony for embezzlement. It still impacts my life now because I'm paying restitution on that felony. It's on my background.

I was doing pretty well for a couple of years. All of a sudden, I'm in a stressful job again. I don't need to go into how I got this job. It was a startup. I knew I needed to get into a startup because they don't do backgrounds. We ran out of money. We got acquired by an established company and it happened that I got in through the back door. I'm in a seat that's pretty stressful. It's high energy. There's a lot of responsibility that goes with it. I'm blessed that I have the best boss with more compassion I could ever ask for. It is stressful and I found myself going home and having a cocktail every night.

I was big into working out for a few years there. When I got into this seat, this role, the working out went by the wayside, because I didn't have time to work out when I needed to get home and make a drink. That was first and foremost for me. Even when I was sick, I was like "I need a drink. I'm going to drink," because it's all that made me feel better. I was a jerk in front of my daughter, who lived with me. She ended up moving out. All the while, I'm like "It must be her." I literally would drink until I was so intoxicated I could not walk. I'd pass out. I would be hung over, but the hangovers totally stopped it. I remember a friend asking me, "You don't drink at work, do you?" I go, "No. If I drink at work, that'd be a problem." All of a sudden, without me even realizing the way my disease was progressing, at this time I did not even believe it was a disease. As far as me drinking, it was an all-evening thing, and that was it. Either I was hung over the next day or I wasn't, but I would drink every night and on the weekends.

Eventually, I would drink in the mornings before I went to work because I felt like a mess. I would drink all day long at work, to a point where I wouldn't even get drunk anymore. I forgot what it felt like to feel good from alcohol. I know it's a cool buzz and all that good stuff in the beginning. Eventually, alcoholism turns into a mess. There's no fun in it. Not for me, anyway. There were no hangovers because I needed it to function. I was eventually completely addicted to alcohol. I would drink vodka straight. No mixers because that was extra calories. I started missing work. I was driving under the influence. I never got caught up. There never was a wakeup call. I was a little bit pressed. My best friend and my sister showed up at my house one morning. It was 9:00 a.m. on a Tuesday, September 11, 2018. They took me to Kaiser because I have Kaiser. I had been drinking for a few days

368

and I'd missed work. My boss knew what was up; he's not stupid. I went to Kaiser with no appointment. We showed up there around 10:30 a.m. and the woman or the doctor or the one who was taking non-appointments (it's called a crisis line or something like that), she comes out, ends up being the person who is the main decision-maker with residential.

I don't even know what it was because I was always drunk. I could basically go to bed, wake up, and go to Kaiser for a CDRP, which I tried before that. I tried outpatient three times. My boss put me through it. I wouldn't go to meetings. It never worked for me. I'd be drunk there or I'd get drunk after. I'd test dirty there. They were pressing for residential. I'm like "No, I can't do that." Finally, it was either that or I was going to probably drink myself to death. I knew that. The doctor who ended up taking those without appointments that morning was the decision-maker for residential. I didn't even have to go through the approval process. It basically was like "I'll call The Camp and I'll call the MPI in Oakland." I remember her saying, "One is a hospital setting and one is outdoors," and I was like "I don't care what they are. I'm hoping that they don't have a bed available for weeks," because I knew it was inevitable, but I was not ready. I wanted to go home and drink. That morning, I'd run out of alcohol, so I did some cocaine that I had left over for months ago. I smoked the rest of my weed. I was pretty lit when I went in there. I didn't even know what was going on. Twenty minutes later, they hadn't even finished taking my vitals and they got a call from The Camp saying there was a bed available. I needed to be there that day by 2:00 in order to check in and get my bed.

I had 25 minutes to pack. I was in total denial. My sister's like "That's all you're going to pack?" I'm like "Yes," thinking I'm not going, I'm not going to waste my time, but I went. I was there. At The Camp is where I learned that addiction is a disease. I never believed that. I thought I was weak. I thought I couldn't handle life, which is true. With the right tools, knowledge and program, if I work it the right way and stay with the right type of people, go to meetings, and do what they say, I can handle life sober. I'm learning that. There wasn't a bed available anywhere when I got out of The Camp Recovery Center. I was there for 45 days. We tried to find one and it wasn't happening right away. I went home. I was okay for a few days. It was a wrap. I missed a day at work, which is crazy because I had gotten back after being gone for a couple of months. I drank all day until I passed out. I wake up, drink more, pass out, wake up, and drink more. This happened all day, Thursday night, Friday, and Saturday. It would have continued through Sunday night. I probably missed work on Monday because that was my routine, but it just so happened I had some sisters who love me.

One was in Gault House and one is at Lotman, and there were girls who I met at The Camp Recovery Center. We only knew each other 30 days and they came all the way to Hayward, picked me up, and brought me out here to Santa Cruz. I got a room at Gault House that Sunday night. I'm forever thankful because that's where I'm at now. I know for a fact I was sick from drinking. If I had stayed home and I would have continued,. I probably would have been

370

hospitalized because I had not been hungover in at least two years because I needed the alcohol to function. I had gone through withdrawals and I had come out of that at The Camp. When I got out, I thought I could drink as much as I could before I went in. It was a no-go because I was ill for at least two days. I have 11 days clean now. I'm grateful. I have my job. It's still the same stress level, but I am coping because I come home to Gault House and I go to meetings every day or evening. My family is supportive. They're proud of me. They're happy. I feel healthy. My kids love being around me. They call me all the time. My life has changed now. I'm thankful.

What did your early recovery look when you were at The Camp?

I felt every emotion that you could possibly feel. The first few days I was a little bit timid. I was taking it all in, not scared, but a little bit. I was soft, where I was nice to everybody. The second week I was happy. I have a problem with people telling me what to do, authority figures, and I have a feeling it's because of the way I was brought up in such a strict home. We had a family weekend the second weekend I was there. It's the tail end of my happy week. My sister and my eldest daughter were there for a family day on Sunday and we had communicated that day. We all talked. About two out of the 12 clients who were in there with their families said they extended. All of a sudden, "Everybody's extending, Mom. You should extend too." I was looking forward to getting out of my 30 days. Also, I don't like things to be other people's idea. I wanted it to be my idea. If I was going to extend, it would be my idea and I didn't like that. It sent me into this depression for a few days. It was turmoil. I could not even be myself. I was unhappy. My sisters were concerned. At The Camp, my counselor got me through it. He lit a fire under me and got me to break down in the process group. We had a process group every day. That's when I came out of that depression and I decided on my own I was going to extend because he said, "Now that you took your mask off; it's time to get to work.

What do you think about the 12-Steps program?

I'm new to the 12-Steps program. I don't even have a sponsor yet. I believe that from what I hear and from knowing what the steps are that everybody should do the 12 Steps. I don't think that it should just be a thing for addicts at all. It makes you a better person, and I look forward to starting the work once I find somebody to do that with.

What does your future look like?

I could go one way, but I won't even entertain that thought. Let's say the sober Andrea—I want to go back to school. I'm in the Legal department at work, and I want to learn everything there is to learn about the legal system and the job that I do, corporate law and in-house council. Anyway, I want to be the best employee; I want to be stellar. My boss is stellar and he deserves a stellar employee. I want to be an awesome mom. I know that both my daughters will one day get married and have their own kids. I want to be an awesome grandmother who's healthy and able to play and has the means to spoil my grandbabies. I'm not married now. I am in a relationship. I don't know where that's going to take me. However, I'm not worried about that. All I'm focused on is my sobriety and my job. Sobriety first, without that, I'd be a mess at work. Unfortunately, my boss knows me now. I can't get by with anything, even if I tried, but I don't want to. It's all about sobriety, but my future looks bright.

Andrea, thank you. To our audience, stay sober and be happy.

8. Billy: Male, 55, Gang Life, Prison, and Meth

Bill is a big African American man from Salinas, California, who started using weed at the tender age of 11. Billy is now 55 years old and he is funny and easy to like. He does stand-up comedy, and until recently, he had to be loaded before he went on stage. Billy snores loudly and it has been difficult to match him with a suitable roommate. He is 55 years old and he has been addicted to crack and meth, as well as alcohol, weed, and a little bit of everything else.

Bill, how are you doing?

I'm blessed to be here. I came a long way. Where did I begin? I'm going to take it from the very beginning. I grew up in Salinas. I grew up during the Cesar Chavez times. It was like a racial thing. Mexican people were mad at that time. They were picketing and my little family was walking through their neighborhood to go to school in the morning, which was a big issue. I would get chased a lot and beat up a lot. I didn't blame the people because they were so angry at the time about things and their madness weren't for us. We were coming through at the wrong time. It changed my life because it forced me to be involved with gangs. I felt like that was my only protection. In my childhood, that's where I go back. I think that it attributed to my addiction too. I remember going to school, and on the way to school, I would get beat up. When I would get to school, I'd be in such bad shape that the teachers wouldn't want to let me go to school.

Sometimes they would catch you and give you a choice, "Either we pee on you, or we beat you up."

My dad was a military man. That was the worst thing in the world as far as his son to come through, coming to school, smelling like pee. It's such a big dishonorable thing. I began to run all the time. I'd run back, but then my brothers are coming up. I remember the turning point of me wanting to be affiliated was they caught my little brother, who I loved so much. They told him, "Billy, I'd rather for them to pee on me than to beat me up." That grabbed me bad. I was like "You can stop this if you're a part of this." The gang at that time to me was so intimidating. I was still a part of the gang. I'll wear blue and that'll keep me safe. It was the greatest two weeks in the world that I wore blue. I was wondering, these Mexican dudes, they don't ever bother dudes who wear blue. The gang caught up with me. Basically, they'd beat the snot out of me and then they said, "You took it good. If you want to be a part of us, we'll be there after school. You should be there." I was like "I went this far." I've been lying to my mom and dad. If they asked what happened to me, I'll say, "I fell down the stairs."

I went to school and I didn't know there was so many of them. They said, "Do you want to be a part of us? Go ahead and choose one of us to beat up." I was looking around; I'm looking for the smallest sucker over there. I did choose him. The minute I swung on him, the whole chapter jumped on me. They basically jumped on me. They said, "You got jumped in. Do you want to be a part of this?" He said,

"You've got to remember that if someone messed with one of us, they mess with all of us."

I'm going through things in my childhood and I'm watching my dad. My dad, he's good about it. He has a drinking problem, but he's keeping it in the closet. Every once in a while, we catch him messed up at parties. I'm at a point where I'm stealing his liquor and drinking it. I'm hanging out with my friends, and I'm getting something for them out of my dad's stash. We're getting drunk.

How old were you at this point?

I was 13 when I was noticing that it was a problem. It carried on until I was about 15 or 16. I would do it because everyone else was doing it, but I really wasn't into it. I didn't like the taste. Some people can drink and eat. I couldn't do that. It was nasty to me. I didn't want to do that. I started smoking weed at that time, which I didn't look at as that bad. I had to hide it. To me, it wasn't that bad. We'd experiment with mushrooms and PCP when we get all rah-rah. That went on and then crack came out and I was selling crack. Crack to me was the forbidden thing. You could sell it, but don't smoke it.

Everybody who I was around at that time who started me off selling it was like "We don't even want you to touch it with your hands." All the people who held me down, it was like a handful of like seeds or dandelions and everybody was holding you down and making you follow the rules and do things. They either got locked up, shot, killed, left, or they testified against somebody. Therefore, they left me with the crack. Me and crack got married. I couldn't enjoy a woman with crack. I was like "You're not putting your mouth on crack and me." It's another mouth to feed. Crack doesn't want this and I don't want this. Me and crack, we need to be together.

It's like a third-wheel thing.

Crack made me break up with my family. Crack made me sell my cars, all my belongings. It was like a cold-blooded, tough spouse. It was really hard. I would go days and I would take, steal, lie, and cheat so much that I forget to remember or remember to forget. I would steal things and mail them back to myself. That's how out of it I was. I would take the envelope with me because I know for a fact I'm going to jack shit. When I run out of crack, I'm jacking something. I would go through so much. I know I'd have so much that I would end up mailing it back to myself. I did that a lot of times and I'd be shocked like "$500? That was cool. I don't even remember how it got here, but it looks like my signature on this." It was bad. I felt like I got made of example because I got caught with $10 worth of crack. Crack at that time was like "You don't want to get caught with crack residue." I got caught with $10 worth of crack on me. They gave me altogether three years. I was like "$10? Black with crack could do it." You go see the penitentiary at that time.

What year was that?

This is like '83. It was quite an experience. It got me deeper and deeper in being affiliated because that's the only way you're going to survive at that time. I got out of that. I ended up doing time there. The minute I got out, I was making up for lost time with my lady and started having kids. I wasn't over with it. I was still putting my family through hell, my wife through hell. She was waiting for me when I got out and it was terrible. I am into a program that helped me, it was Genesis House. I remember that was a turning point in my life. I went to Genesis House and then it was like an attack program to the point where you would act out different scenarios.

I'm fresh out of prison and I go to this program. I'm in there with 13 women and this other guy. We find out that these women are all prostitutes. It was hard. My first day in the program, I came in there with braids. I'm buff. The coordinator, the manager of the place, she's talking to me and finding out where I am, talking to my parole officer and everything, and she sums me up and says, "You've got a real macho problem. That's what's wrong with you. You think you're a He-Man or Hercules." That's what she said. I was like "I don't like her off the top. She's putting me in a category like this."

She comes back, and she goes, "What I want you to do is pick out colors in this box and then you're going to draw a sign." I'm like "All right." I actually picked out blue and black, and she goes, "You picked them out?" I was like "Yes." She

378

goes, "Those are the affiliation-gang colors. That's not going to work." She goes and gives me a pink pen to draw a sign with, which bent me over. I don't even like the color pink to draw stuff with, and she's like "You're going to make a sign that says, "I am not as macho as I think." I said, "I'm not going to do that." She goes, "I can call your parole officer because you're not going along with this program." I was like "I'm not as macho as I think." She was hard. They would do car washes. I was doing this in Seaside, which is that far from where I grew up. A lot of people in Seaside I had rivals with. They would see me with the pink sign that says, "I am not as macho as I think." We had to do car washes. I had to get used to it.

How long did you have to wear the sign for?

It was a contract. It was from 9:00 to 5:00. That was a tough thing. I couldn't wait to take it off at the end of the day and then the next day it would start again. After a while, it really didn't bother me. I got over that and they could see I got over that. I was counseling other people when they come into the program. You're able to see a lot of people that come in who have the same problem that you might have. It's like this right here, that you're able to help other people. To me, part of my sobriety, part of getting better, was being able to help someone else. One of the things that I like to do is to give back.

I didn't graduate that program. I can't make excuses, but it was hard coming from prison and then to living with 13 prostitutes. It was a tough thing because interviewing them—some of the stories that they would tell me and the other dude. We're interviewing them. Some of the stories that they would tell about what happened to them, I think they would make it erotic on purpose. It was hard to focus on your program or try to help somebody when you're like "This woman is something. I'm sorry about what happened, but what happened in the shower?" It was a tough thing and it helped me get off of crack. After a while, I got done with that, and I got back with my ex-wife, and she stuck with me a lot. She went beyond the call. Some of the things I would put her through, I thought that she would have left me. I would have actually left me.

Did she have a drug problem at all?

I would not let her. She didn't even ask that many times, but it seemed like she asked me a lot. She wanted to be on the same level as me if she's going through everything that I did. She was pregnant with my first son. I was like the dirt on the bottom of your shoe, but I cannot let that happen. Maybe that's being stingy or selfish, but I couldn't let her do it.

It's the opposite of being stingy or selfish. I recognize some of it might be you want it for yourself. Also, you care about her. I think it can be both. You don't want to see her get to where you're at.

Yeah, but when you're on crack, all that is quickly thrown out of the window.

380

You're focused on that rock.

Yes. I remember when I used to sell it I'd be seeing so many terrible things. People were giving up their food stamps. Kids were waiting outside the dope house waiting for their mom to come out. "When you go in there, could you see my mom? She has food stamps." The worst thing about it is you're the one who got the food stamps from her, which is her baby's food. It's like you have no morals. You don't care. It's only about you. It's a cold-blooded piece. I would not let her do crack. After that portion, I didn't complete the program, but I got a lot out of it. From there, I started doing construction work and doing positive things. From there, I started doing private security work, working as a bouncer, and that was another thing that caused me to be around alcohol a lot. At first it was no big deal. I didn't believe in being drunk and trying to force somebody at a bar to leave because they were acting like a fool, because they were drunk.

I would feel like I was righteous because I would wait until the bar was closed and everybody's gone. We're there and that's when I would get drunk. For the most part, drinking to me is like snoring. It was like "I don't think it's that bad of a problem," but to the people sleeping next to you in the same house, that's a problem. You need to fix that. I'm thinking, they could be lying on me. My throat's a little dry. Maybe I could snort a little bit. I would get drunk so bad that I would actually go and look for my car in the morning. The first thing I do is ask, "Where did I leave my car?"

I remember one time I was thinking ahead and I hid the car from me. I'm almost scared to call the police because there's probably open liquor inside that car. It's a tough thing. I got to the point where if I go out and drink, I'm not going to drive. If I wasn't working, I get hammered. I got to the point where I didn't want to get that drunk and I found cocaine would take you out of the drunkenness. It almost erases you being drunk and like "Let's giddy-up. Let's ride doors." I started doing stand-up comedy, which is a thing that I've found where I almost think that I would be forgiven if I could make people laugh. There's a sickness in that. I almost feel I'd be forgiven about a lot of things if I can make people laugh for the wrongs that I did to them. Laughter is a very powerful thing.

I'm going to fast-forward to where I got injured really bad. I got bit by a brown recluse spider. I'd take a shower and the skin would literally fall off. The doctors started giving me Oxycontin. And I was like "I couldn't feel pain when he gave me the Oxies. I don't feel anything." I was like "This is a good feeling." It's a good feeling until they don't give it to you anymore. I remember, it was almost like he was saying in slow motion, "I can't refill this for you anymore." I intimidated him so badly when he said I couldn't have it that they call the security on me. I was upset. You know how you have it in your mind like "I'll talk to you later. Let me get my Oxycontin and I'll be right back with you." There's nothing. I was like "You're going to need help for this right here. You're going to need some help." It's like saying, "We're going to stop you from drinking water. You're not going to get more water."

Especially, when you already expect it, I know what you mean. It's already right there in front of you and then all of a sudden, it's not.

You hate him. It was a tough piece. They called security on me and I came back again. I was more or less hunting him and saying, "Give me one more and we'll call it even right there. I'm not going to bother you anymore. I don't even like doctors." That didn't work out. The only thing I can find is that I'm going to have to be my own pharmacy, my own prescription thing, because this pain is too much. This pain is going to put me in jail and they aren't going to give me any good pain medication in jail. I'm going to have to go out there and get my own medication. Meth took away the pain. I was shocked at meth. I'm like, "I don't feel anything. I should go put my track shoes on. This is stupendous."

I wasn't shooting it. I was smoking it and I would make a meth chewing gum. I was putting it in everything, putting it in a cigarette, saying, "Let's smoke meth in a joint." A lot of people would smoke weed with me, thinking this is some good-ass weed. I was like "You just smoked meth and you didn't even know it." It's the same way with my weed pipe. "Let me smoke," and then they'd be following that. It was terrible and I didn't care. It's like that with crack. I didn't care who I got hooked. I was terrible. I remember telling this woman that what she was smoking was a blonde hash. "Don't even worry about it. It's good." That's wrong. They start following you. It's like "Where did you get this hash at?" "I might know a guy."

I'm getting high on meth, but I wasn't high enough until I could feel like ghosts and spirits are following me. That's when I was like "This is where I want to be at, trying to dodge some devils." It would keep me up for three or four days. It was making me worse. When I come down, I would feel everything. I scratched a hole in my skin and the hole was getting bigger. I don't know if meth was getting on it and making it bigger. I would get so high and drunk I would start scratching a big open wound. I remember going to the hospital and they were like "What are you doing?" I was like "There was something in there. I had to get it out." It was bad. I'll sleep with my girlfriend and I end up bleeding in the bed really bad, which is a turn-off. It was hard to get back in bed with your whole leg hemorrhaging, plus you bleed in the bed, doubled over in pain. That's going to be the no-no. Our relationship went on the rocks right then.

I began to get homeless. I was like "Things have gotten worse. Do you know what's wrong with you? You need some more meth. That's what's wrong with you," all this thinking. I got to the point where I'm sleeping on the beach and I'm sleeping in the woods. I was able to handle that. I got that big Grizzly Adams type nature thing. I'm cool with that until I got poison oak in my wound. I got a big open wound on my leg, and when I'm not high, I could barely walk. I'm getting high all the time because I'd do anything not to feel that pain. It's bad. When I get so high, I start scratching the wound. I'm like "These are cheap socks. I've got to get some better socks. It can't even hold a little blood. I saw a lot of blood coming out of your leg there."

384

I ended up going to the hospital again. I had so many days where I go to the hospital that it was accumulating. There, each one of them say, "This is not good. You need to get off your leg and rest it." I'm like "Like I'm going to do that. Where am I going to rest it? On a park bench?" My options were few. It got to the point where my ex-girlfriend felt bad for me and she's like "I know you're going through hell right now. You can come and stay here." She let me stay over there and made sure I was going to the hospital and whatnot. I have to still do comedy. That's the only thing I got that's making me not feel so depressed. It's going out doing shows. When I do comedy, it's like I have a different persona. When I get up on the stage, I'm like this cocky black dude who isn't scared of nothing. After I get down, I'm so drunk because I need that before I get up on stage.

To all the people who I bounced out of a club, I was like this tough guy, but now I'm doing stand-up comedy. It's like a weird metaphor. I can't understand it. I ended up catching a case because this guy would not leave me alone and I assaulted him bad. They gave me two years in prison for that. It was nothing more than a bar fight outside, but it's all the racks against me before. I was ex-affiliated. I was an ex-gang member and I sold crack back in the days. They made me do two years altogether in prison for that, which was like a wake-up to be wounded badly in the lion's den. That's the best I could explain it.

Did they give you treatment at least when you were locked up?

They really didn't believe at first that I was hurt that bad until they'd seen it. They said, "We're not going to give you anything but some Tylenol in here." I was like "Okay." The pain would get so bad that I'm kicking Oxycontin and I'm kicking meth. They ended up putting me in a special little wing in there all by myself. No roommate is getting to rest with me. We're going to war. I'm kicking, plus I'm wounded. I'm in pain, and everything's bothering me. They put me in solitary. Jesus and I started doing time together. That's basically it. God and I started doing time together. Everything around me needed a break from me. That's probably what it was.

Everything around me needed a break from Bill. Even my mom needed a break. My family needed a break. I could totally understand that now it was a crusher. I was like, "Nobody is coming to see me. No one? I didn't think I was that bad." There again, it was like I was snoring. I didn't think it was that bad, but people thought it was terribly bad. I ended up going to San Quentin. I'm not giving the prison system all these props, but I ended up doing time over it. I got out and I went to New Life Treatment Center here in Santa Cruz. New Life was good to me. It took me a while to get used to things, but I thank God for them. I think that when it gets down to it, you being sober, you have to make up your mind to do it. I've been sober for years, but I can't attribute it to "I've made up my mind and I decided I'm not going to do it." That's BS.

The law said, "Snoring man, we're going to lock you up." Sometimes life and things come into play where you could never think you're that bad. You can never feel like it's time for me to put the pipe away and back away from it. I'm one of the people who I have to get pointed in the right direction. I'm not getting it. I'm totally wrong. I do snore. I'm one of those people. I'm working on that and I even go to a lot of meetings and I don't try to get chips. I want to have a year on my own sober, not to be force-fed it because it's a good thing. I think it's a good thing, but I want that on my own. I want to own it.

I totally understand where you're coming from, but I would almost counter. When you were at New Life, perhaps even in prison, but certainly at New Life, you could have walked away and bought a bottle or a bag or whatever. You didn't do it. You have done drunks or alcohol while you've been here. You have still done this. You mentioned Jesus or God. Perhaps it's with your higher power's help. You're still making that decision to "not use." I would encourage you to at least own that and recognize that for whatever and however you're doing it, you have made the decision to stay sober and that's huge, especially compared to how it sounds like it was before.

I was terrible and then not being able to see it. Knowing how to call it quits is the thing. "Call it quits. What's wrong with you, Bill? You need to get some more drugs in you. That's what's wrong with you. That's why you have this second fight. You've got to quit rehab. Mr. Sir, you need to go ahead and get some good shot and get you a good toke, and then see if you want to quit." I never did get it until right now.

I can see things don't affect me and get at me like they used to you. Maybe it's because I'm older. I am a bit older, but I can see where I'm going and I like what I'm doing.

I like feeling like I don't need to go and do that. I don't need to go pay for that. I don't need to find him so he can get me some of this right here. I like waking up in the morning time, knowing where my vehicle is at. I like waking up in the morning time and going to my job and meaning something. It's a good feeling. I'm not rich or anything, but I can see how far I've come from and that's a good feeling. Knowing that your family and your people want you around, they can't wait for you to come around, compared to where they couldn't wait for you to leave. It's a big difference. I'm blessed in that.

I don't want to be a sore winner, but I'm feeling good about this. As far as my sobriety, I know I'm running toward it and trying to do this. A lot of times I go back and I think about how long I was on drugs compared to before that I wasn't doing them and the two don't compare. I've always done either weed, alcohol, or some type of drug. It's hard to sum up. It's hard to admit that you wasted a lot of time, you wasted a lot of years. You've made a lot of people unhappy. You've done so many bad things. If I can sum it up, it's because I want to do better. That might sound weak or not the answer, but I want to do a lot better.

I wouldn't say that sounds weak. I think that's the opposite. That sounds strong, especially if that's what motivates you. I'm the same way. I gave a lot of years to my addiction, but now we get to give a lot of years to our recovery. I admit, it's hard not to look at those mistakes as failures or a waste of time, but it's a learning experience. If that can inform you about who we are now and then the choices we make from here on out, I think it's valuable. I like that analogy you use of the snoring and not being able to see it. Like our addiction, we can't see how bad it is. What are your hopes for the future from here on out?

My hopes are to be able to make a path, so someone else can walk in and see which way to go. Maybe even counsel, even be able to give back and do a program and help somebody. There's one thing about being a dope fiend or ex-dope fiend, you can tell a lot of times which people and the problems they go through, you can understand it. You see where they might need some nurturing here or being able to draw back and see "Am I just pouring water on a dead flower? Do they want this too?" I think a lot of times if you put the energy out, it's like when you went to go get your dope, you didn't even care. It's like "I'm going to do this. It's going to go down. If I have to go to a different county or a bad neighborhood, I'm going to go ahead and make this happen." That's what I've got to do and people have to do with their sobriety. You have to take no days off and go get it.

I want to thank you, Bill, for joining us here today. To all our readers, we wish you to stay sober and to be happy.

9. Heather: Female, 28, Cocaine at the District Attorney's office

Heather is 28 years old and has been addicted to cocaine and alcohol. Heather is from Sacramento, California, and has 40 days of clean time.

Congratulations and welcome to the interview, Heather.

Thank you.

How did your addiction start?

I was born in Glendale, Arizona, and adopted by my parents, who are from Sacramento, California. I had a good upbringing. My parents gave me anything and everything I could ever have wanted and set a good example for me. Throughout high school, I never partied. I never did anything. I was a good girl. Right after graduating from high school, I was 17 years old and my mom got diagnosed with breast cancer right before her fiftieth birthday. In going through that, taking her to her doctor's appointments, seeing her sick as a dog, I didn't want to see that. I didn't want to feel that anymore. I started off with smoking a little bit of pot here and there. That got rid of these feelings and it led to going out and drinking. I was always a blackout drinker. I drank until I blacked out. I was the one at the party who's making a fool of themselves, not remembering what they did the next day, passed out on the lawn. Not attractive at all.

Soon after that, I got involved with cocaine and all of that to bring me out of my shell, but still not wanting to feel those feelings, even after my mom went through treatment.

Even at home, before I was 21, I was allowed to have wine with my parents. That was always acceptable in the house. They never knew about my cocaine addiction. They knew I smoked pot every once in a while, but not very often. I turned 21 and I had a job. I thought everything was under control. I was going out to the bars every single night until 2:00 a.m., drunker than a skunk, calling my parents to come pick me up or even driving myself home, which scares me to death now.

I was getting up and going to work the next day. I thought my life was still manageable. I still had everything going for me. I got involved in the medical field. I had been doing that for the last 10 years because of my mom, when she was going through breast cancer, that's what prompted me to go into the medical field.

In 2013, I had a day off work and went to my doctor's appointment in the morning, and at 10:30 in the morning on my way home, I was T-boned by a drunk driver. At that same time, I was moving away from my hometown. At 23 years old, that's hard to lose all of your so-called friends, even though they weren't actually friends, just people I got loaded with. I learned that very quickly when you're down, you're out. You have nothing and you need people there for you. I can't walk, I can't drive, I can't even shower or change by myself. I need help and nobody's there for me. These people that you thought were your friends are not there for you. That was hard on me.

I started drinking more, taking pain pills along with it. Surprisingly, I never continued down that road of pills, which I'm thankful for now. I was at the time of using them heavily. Alcohol was my main escape. That was my way to forget about everything. In a sense, it was like when I blacked out, I didn't remember. It never happened, forget about it, don't worry about it, and keep rolling on.

In going through my physical recovery from my car accident, I got a settlement from the accident and I bought my own house. That's when my addiction picked up. I was by myself and drink by myself, used by myself. No one knew what I was doing or how much or how frequent. It started with a couple of bottles of wine a night. Then I would go to the store and buy another one, calling in sick to work a lot, coming up with all these excuses. I worked for this wonderful company, a private practice. I messed it up. I did. I called in sick often. I was buying a lot more cocaine and they go hand-in-hand because the more cocaine I did, the more I could drink.

I was detaching from my family, from my friends, isolating myself. My high school sweetheart would tell me, "You're an alcoholic. You drink too much." Hiding the cocaine behind his back and not telling him that I was doing that, I knew I could get away with it. Who's going to think? I had met a new guy. We started dating and moved in together about eight months after dating. He's an addict as well; he's into pills. Again, that's not my thing. It's not what draws me in. He took care of me financially. I was able to use my money for my drug of choice, drinking every day. If I had a good day, I would drink.

If I had a bad day, I would drink. Anything to drink every single day, that's what I did.

I had fallen off cocaine for a little while and got back into it. He was doing it with me. I was doing more than he knew. I had our dealer and then my own personal dealer. It was so messed up. I was that person who hid things all around the house. I had my baggy in my pocket. I had my baggy under the couch pillow cushion. I had my baggy in the bathroom, my baggy in the bedroom. Wherever I was, I could have my fix and he never knew. Until I came here, I finally admitted to how much I was using.

At that same time, I had left my job in the medical profession. I got a job with the District Attorney's office in Sacramento. I was using there. I brought it to work. Again, who's going to think I am using at work? I never thought anybody would ever know and nobody did. I was doing lines in the bathroom. Then I'd come out and talk to the officers like it was no big deal.

That was a good job, solid benefits. I had it going for me. I had my condo still. I was living with my boyfriend in West Sacramento. I just let my house go. I wasn't paying my property taxes, I wasn't paying my bills. It was all going up my nose.

At that time, I didn't care. I didn't care because I was so deep in my addiction, I didn't care about work, I didn't care about my family, I didn't care about my house—my house was going into foreclosure. Thank God, my mom stopped by my condo and saw the sign on the door. It makes me feel terrible because my parents did nothing to deserve what I put them through. They bailed me out.

I quit my job and didn't tell them. I didn't tell my boyfriend. I would get up in the morning and get ready, pretend like I was going to work. I would go do coke all day. Sit in my car, go to the park, hang out. Go to the bars, drink, do coke.

My drinking started to get bad too. I would go out with my friends, and at one point, I went out with my good friend from high school. We went out, we got into a fight, and I walked off. We were in downtown Sacramento. I was blacked-out drunk. Thank God I called one of my mom's friends, and she called my mom, who then called my boyfriend. I told him I was getting an Uber home and he had to drive around downtown Sacramento and find me on the sidewalk with a homeless man taking care of me.

This man was an angel. He had six children, six girls of his own. I could have been raped. I could have been killed. My higher power and my angels were watching over me that night. I don't know how many times they continue to watch over me. They do and they saved my ass so many times. That didn't stop me.

I tried to stop drinking for a month. I was still smoking weed every day, still doing cocaine. I thought I was clean. I wasn't drinking. I was good. I was doing it. Then it started again. "Why can't I have one glass of wine?" That led to two glasses of wine at night and then I was back to the bottles. Wine was my drink of choice and that's what I always drink. Then when I would go out, it would be shots of whiskey and then that's it. Call it a night. Give me a wheelchair; you can't do anything. I'm done.

I've known I needed help for a long time. I didn't want to admit it and I didn't want to stop. I wasn't ready. I pretended like I was going to work. I got up, I got ready. I went out. I had lunch, sitting at the bar, and made friends at the bar, drinking, shots, the whole thing. I got my car and drove across the parking lot where I would meet my dealer. I parked my car and fell asleep in my car. They had to do a wellness check on me. They didn't know if I was alive or if I was dead. I came out of my blackout in an ambulance. Then I came too again and I was in the hospital with my boyfriend standing over me saying, "How did you get here?" My answers were always "I don't know." I can't ever answer the question of what happened or how I got there

My parents and all my loved ones, they don't get the answers that they want either. I stopped drinking again. I was still smoking weed. I was still doing cocaine. That lasted about two weeks. I was trying to go to AA meetings, but I would drink before I went to an AA meeting. I would have a glass of wine so I could walk through the door and be comfortable going in there. I still raise my hand, "Heather, alcoholic, three days. What are you doing? You had a glass of wine." That's how much I did not want to stop. I didn't want to stop at all.

Again, I drank and blacked out and that night I told my mom. She came and picked me up, and I said, "Tomorrow, I need help. Tomorrow, I am going to recover. I need to go to rehab. I need to go to inpatient." I woke up that next morning and she was like "Do you remember what you said last night?" She was like "You wanted to go to rehab. Do you still want to go?" I said, "Yes, I need to go. I've used up all my nine lives. I can't risk my life anymore. I'm going to lose everything."

I almost lost my house. My parents were ready to throw their hands up and say that they were done. My boyfriend was ready to say he was done. I've done all these terrible things to these people who don't deserve it. I made the phone call to the Beacon House Recovery Center. They got me in that day by the grace of God. I'm so thankful that I was willing and that I was ready. I can't live my life like that anymore.

I have 40 days clean today and I can proudly say that is the longest clean time I've ever had. I've never had clean time ever. I'm so excited. I love this person that I am. I truly do. I don't hear that negative self-talk anymore, which says, "You're fat. You're ugly. You're not worth it. You don't deserve it." I never thought that would happen. I look in the mirror and I love myself. I'm so happy with who I am now. I know what I want to do with my future. My recovery is the most important thing in my life. I'm thankful for Gault House, for keeping my ass in check. I need that. I need structure because without that I would go off.

I knew I couldn't go back to Sacramento. If I did, I'd be on the phone. I'd be calling my dealer. I know I would be. To admit that to myself is huge to me. I'm here. I'm looking for a job. My mom came out to visit me and she's so proud of me. I'm happy and excited to start to rebuild that trust. I know it's going to take a long time to get there. All I can do is show her and prove to both of my parents where I'm at and what I'm working toward.

I am taking this seriously and asking for help and reaching out when I need it, though I hate asking for help. I hate it. It's a sign of weakness, but I'm also realizing that it is a strength. It takes a lot of balls to say "I need help. I'm going through some crap and I want to use."

I told my mom if I didn't stop where I was and come here I'd either be in jail or I'd be dead. I'm in the right spot and I thank God every single day for that. He works miracles in ways that I never could imagine. I'm truly blessed.

Tell me what's your opinion of the 12-Step program?

I'm looking for a sponsor. I am going back and forth. I'm having a struggle with doing the NA or AA thing. I'm going to both meetings and there are things that I like in both. I have a lady in AA who I want to ask to be my sponsor. I have a lady in NA that I want to ask to be my sponsor and I'm trying to figure that out. I want to work the steps. I truly do. They're going to help me.

I have a family member who's in recovery. She has more than two years of sobriety under her belt. She's working the steps. She has a sponsor. She has sponsorees. Seeing her succeed is making me want to succeed and go through those. Being able to admit my wrongs and work through those and apologize to the people who I've hurt, to be honest with myself and with other people. I've got to do it.

What do you think works in recovery?

Having that support system, being able to ask for help, admit when I'm wrong, and have no shame in where I've come from. I can only move up. I saw this quote and I can't quite think of it, but it said something along the lines of "It's okay to be knocked down if you pick yourself back up." I'm picking myself up. People get down, but you have to get back up.

I pray every day before my feet hit that ground that I'm not going to use now. I have to take it, day by day, and use the tools that I've learned through prayer and meditation, planting my feet on the floor, remembering where I came from, using that support system, and keeping it going. That's all you can do 10 minutes at a time, even five minutes at a time. You have to take it slow.

I have one last question for you. What does your future look like to you?

My future is happy. My future is clean and sober. My future is having good people around me. I want to be a mother so badly and that could have never happened in my addiction. I could barely take care of myself, let alone take care of another human being. I'm learning how to take care of myself and become an adult.

My future is bright. I would like a career in the medical field and years of sobriety. I would like to help people and giving back to people who helped me or even to people who didn't help me. Being a part of the recovery community, I love that family feeling that you get. You're not alone at all. I was so ashamed. I was so embarrassed to raise my hand and say, "Heather, alcoholic addict." When I hear these people talk, it's all the same. I want to give back to all those people who have helped me continuously every day and push me through those hard times and lift me up when I'm down, being of service and giving back to my community.

Thank you so much. You are a blessing to us here at Gault House. I am so grateful for you and thank you so much for joining us and sharing your story of addiction. To our readers, we wish you to stay sober and happy.

Thank you.

10. Amanda, Female, 26, Alcohol and Cocaine, Spiral of Addiction

Welcome, Amanda.

Thanks for having me.

How did you get started with drug use?

My drug use started in high school. It was mostly drinking before any other harder drugs. The first person I drank with was one of my next-door neighbors. He was older. He graduated from high school. I think that I was 14. My parents drank when I was younger to the point where I saw that they had a problem. I had no inclination to drink at a younger age because of that. I think it was my fourteenth birthday and there were some people hanging out in my neighbor's garage. He made some margaritas and that was my first drink. It started from there and progressed very quickly to the point where I didn't even realize how bad it was.

How much were you drinking?

At the end of my drinking days, I was drinking probably a fifth of Jameson or vodka, whatever was handy, and also doing a good amount of cocaine. I was also smoking marijuana daily.

What size is a fifth?

It's 750 milliliters and I would drink it in one sitting. I was never a morning drinker. My drinking would go on until the wee hours of the night, but I never woke up and drank. I definitely woke up and would do a line of cocaine to kick-start my day. At the end of my drinking, I was bartending. I would go in to work at 4:30 and I wouldn't get off until 2:00. After that, I would go to my friends' houses or I would go back to my place and I'd always have alcohol there. Cocaine is just something that comes with the restaurant industry and something that comes with partying. When you enjoy drinking as much as I did, you don't want to stop and cocaine helps you to keep going. That's how that addiction started.

I knew I was getting in trouble when all of the money I was making on my shift was gone when I woke up in the morning. It was all going to alcohol and drugs. It was a slippery slope and very quickly I had gone over the edge. I got really deep, really fast. By the time I realized how bad it was, it seemed like it was too late because I couldn't back out of it.

How old were you when you first started using cocaine?

I first started using cocaine when I was 21 years old. The job that I worked at, that's something that everyone—all my coworkers—were doing. On Friday nights, there was a karaoke night. There was a crowd of people that I would hang out with once I got off of work that were using it religiously. I had no interest in it because I knew that I would like it and then it got to the point where everyone was just telling me, "Just do one line. Just try it." I was like "I'll try it. I'll do one line." After that first line, I did not stop. At first, it was like "I did that." We partied that night, and then I woke up in the morning hating myself.

That was one of the worst feelings, waking up with a cocaine hangover. After that, I probably didn't do it for a few weeks. All of sudden, I realized that everywhere I went, it was always around me. It was really easy to get. It was fairly expensive, but it wasn't too expensive to the point where I couldn't afford it. I was making really good money bartending. It went from once every few weeks to once a week to twice a week to every day, spending all of my money on it.

Where did you grow up?

I grew up in Santa Cruz, born and raised.

You started drinking at the age of 15 and you started cocaine at the age of 21. You had five years approximately of just drinking. How deep did your alcoholism get? You were saying you were a fifth a day, was that seven days a week?

At the end, yes, that was within the last year, when I was 23 to 24. That's how bad it got. In high school, I really didn't drink that much. I played softball and volleyball all throughout middle school and high school and I even played a little bit in college. I didn't drink that much in high school because my schedule didn't really allow it. I was playing year-round softball competitively. I was playing Fall Ball and then in high school during the spring. During the summer, I played travel ball. I went all over the United States. I've been to Arizona, Utah, Hawaii, Texas, all over, playing. My schedule didn't really allow it. My drinking was sporadic. It would be on spring break or weekends every once in a while.

It wasn't something that was habitual for me until I turned about 19 or 20. Once I graduated from high school—I was going to Cabrillo, which is the local junior college—I tried out for the softball team and I made it. I met a group of older girls who knew everybody and liked to party.

That was a way for me to socially fit in and socially make friends. There was a lot of anxiety going from high school to college. In high school, especially being from Santa Cruz and having an older brother who's one grade higher than me—he's 21 months older than me, but only one grade higher. That was my way throughout my whole life to make friends—it was through him. I always had a built-in friend through him. Also, the fact that he had his whole group of friends, I clung to that.

When I went to Cabrillo, I was on my own for the first time, in some sense of the word. I met these girls and they really liked to party. I had enjoyed alcohol, so I thought that that was the next logical progression. I ended up not doing very well in school at all, not completing classes and getting pushed through just because I played sports. My priority was no longer myself or school or even softball. My priority was drinking and fitting in with these girls and socializing with the cute guys on the baseball team and trying to find out what the next best thing was going to be.

This was at the age of 19 and 20, and then you became a bartender. I'm assuming you had to be 21 to become a bartender, is that correct?

That's correct. I started out as a host at this restaurant and then quickly went to bussing. I moved to Long Beach for a year when I was 20 with a guy who I had met and didn't know that long. It was my first relationship that the drinking played a huge role in. He was a little bit older than me. We didn't know each other that long, but I wanted to get out of Santa Cruz. I was bored. I was stagnant. I didn't have any inclination or anything holding me here.

He wanted to get out as well, so we ended up moving to Long Beach together. It was a volatile relationship from the beginning because we never knew each other. All we did was party together, and mistakes were made by both of us. I turned to drinking and turned to marijuana. I didn't use any cocaine in Long Beach but turned definitely to the social aspect of drinking because I felt very alone down there. I didn't know anybody, and we weren't getting along. It was just not a good situation. He ended up staying. Once I came back from Long Beach, I went back to the restaurant and I had just turned 21. I started cocktail serving and then eventually started bartending. When I turned 21 and came back, the party was on. It was a nonstop party from there. I didn't even attempt to go back to school. I had no goals, no aspirations. My only goal was to have as much fun as I possibly could. I did have fun for a little while until it got to the point where it was unmanageable.

You came back, and you were bartending, and you were 21. The cocaine started, which assisted you to drink more and stay up later. The parties became longer and heavier. Did you get into any drugs after cocaine?

I've tried Molly (Ecstasy) a number of times. I thoroughly enjoy it, but that was one of those things, with the emotional hangover, that was far too much for me to handle. It drains everything in you. I was so depressed that I should have decided to leave everything behind. I decided that that was not something that meshed well with me. I decided I didn't need to use that anymore, and I had other things that made me feel fine.

Was it perhaps your first introduction to the concept of saying no to a particular product?

It was the only concept I've ever had of saying no to a mind-altering substance. That was the only time that I can really remember saying no to anything because everything made me feel great for the moment.

On your cocaine usage, let me ask a little bit about the quantities that you were using so the reader might be able to get some bearing on what quantities we are talking about and how much money you were spending on it. Can you talk to that point?

At first, I was never buying the cocaine. I was hanging around the people who had it. I had no idea of how much it costs. When it got to the point where I wanted to do it by myself and I didn't want to share it with anyone, I was going through at least a half gram to a gram a night. A gram cost's about $70 if it's not very good. It's upwards of that depending on how good it is. I never found anything that was really as good as the first stuff I did. I think that's more of a mind trick.

About $100 a day and was that seven days a week?

It was whenever I could get it, whenever I tried to get it. At that time, I was working about six days a week. There wasn't a shift toward the end that I didn't go to work with some in my pocket.

What are some of the worst experiences you can describe while you were using?

Embarrassment and humiliation—there have been a few times when I have done things for people in order to get cocaine. There have been times when I put myself in risky situations knowing they're risky because I wasn't done with the party, my night wasn't over. There have been people who have taken advantage of me when I wasn't in a coherent state.

Why do you think that you were using drugs at all?

It's always been a social thing for me. I don't have much problem talking to people of the opposite sex, or of the same sex. I always thought that that's what you did socially. For me, it was self-justification of how you make friends as an adult. Once you get to 21—that's why the drinking age is 21, because that's what you do. That's what I was doing for a really long time. I was born and raised in Santa Cruz. I can tell you exactly what the inside of every bar looks like, but I can't tell you what every beach looks like or what our national forest looks like.

It was also the environment that I was around. Had I not been bartending and had I not surrounded myself with people who did that, then I don't think that this is the path that I would have taken. If I would have taken my priorities a little bit more seriously or my interest even more seriously, rather than other people's interests, then I think that my life would have gone a much different route. I'm grateful to be here. This is the best mind state that I've been in in a very long time. Sometimes you have to go through the trenches to get to the other side. That's where I am now.

You seem to be in a pretty good space to me. You're also young, so if you went down some wrong roads, you realized it fairly quickly. You can choose which roads you want to go down in the future. The roads that you've been down in the past are not dictating which roads you want to go down in the future. I want to give you some assurances that you're doing just fine.

Thank you. I'm lucky to have an amazingly supportive family that was there and has had my back through this whole journey that I'm on. All I had to do was ask for help one time and all of them moved mountains for me. I'm very grateful and I'm very blessed to have everyone in my life that I do.

One of the things that I feel I want to say as a way of trying to be supportive to you is to tell you that the desire to be liked is an Achilles' heel. You were talking about your motivation for using drugs as largely social. To me, it sounds like you want to be liked, which most people do, but it's an Achilles' heel and it comes with consequences. I'm not sure if that's a good aspiration in the first place. I'd like to focus on the turning point. I'm thinking there was a mental process that happened inside you or there was some significant external event that happened but there was a turning point where you decided to ask for help and seek help. Can I ask you to talk about that turning point?

I was at a wedding with my mom in Carmel. I had stayed up all night the night before, well knowing that this wedding's been planned for over a year. We had RSVP'd over a year prior to this and I had known that this date was coming. I chose to stay up all night. I didn't sleep at all. I showed up late and my mom was perturbed about that. We drove over there. On the way over there, I stopped at a gas station to get gas, went in, and got two little shot-sized pings of Fireball, and pounded those, and then got back in the car. We got to the wedding and I had some cocaine left over from the night before. We walked into the wedding and I walked straight into the bathroom and did a line, then went and hung out with my mom the whole time. It was fun. It was a really great time. We were drinking the whole time. My mom doesn't drink like an alcoholic, though she enjoys drinking. We've had a rocky past, she and I. At this point or previously, me being 24 years old and on my own, she saw drinking as something that I enjoyed and that was something we could connect over and that's something that we could do together because she didn't really realize how bad I had gotten.

We were drinking at the wedding and then we went back to the hotel. We're drinking there, and I was drinking and doing cocaine. My mom looked at me and she was like "You've had like 15 drinks. How are you, okay? How are you still talking and not slurring your words? How are you still standing upright?" We went back to the room and I broke down and I was like "I've been doing loads of cocaine and I need help. I don't know how to stop using alcohol and drugs, and I feel like I'm lost. I don't know where I'm going, but I know it's not a good place."

We sat there, and we cried. I could see the pain in her eyes. I don't want to say that she was disappointed, but I think that she was willing to do anything to help me. She felt sad that I had felt so desperate all this time and wasn't able to reach out and ask for help. We woke up in the morning and drove back to Santa Cruz. She had called a bunch of places the night before and said that she found a bed for me at The Camp Recovery Center in Scotts Valley. I drove straight to my job and quit. We went to my house. She moved all of my stuff out of my house and I was in treatment.

What were the causes of you having a difficult relationship with your mother prior to this because she was the one you went to and confessed to? Mothers being mothers are always there for their children. Did you have typical daughter-mother issues?

My parents always had a tumultuous relationship with each other. They never thoroughly enjoyed being around each other. I have an older brother and a younger brother. There's never been a day that all three of us went without hearing "I love you" from both of them and getting big hugs. They really didn't enjoy being around each other, however. I think seeing that made me want to grow up a lot faster than I should have. I've seen them not be very nice to each other and be generally unhappy with their own lives because they felt like they had to stay together for us. When I was 15, my parents got a divorce. That took a toll on all of us. I don't think that I realized this when my drinking started. It just coincided. That's the time in my life where I decided that I wanted to start drinking. That's what we were doing. It wasn't that I was heartbroken over my parents finally getting a divorce; I was ecstatic that they were because immediately I saw the change in them. They seemed a lot happier.

Because of all the years of me having to follow them around and pick up the pieces a little bit, I grew up a lot faster than my parents wanted me to or that I needed to. My mom and I would always clash really hard because I always was trying to play the parent. I was always trying to be older than I was. I was always trying to kind of parent her and parent my father and try to separate them like they were fighting siblings. That's where the relationship between her and I got rocky.

It stayed that way throughout high school until I was 18. When I was 18, I moved out into my first apartment with a few girls I had met. After that, with a little distance put between us, I realized how much she was doing for me and doing for all of us. That made me a little more grateful, as I should have been the whole time. Being 16, 17, and 18 are hard ages for a girl. I took that out on her and she wasn't having it, so she pushed back. That would create us to push against each other.

That's where it stemmed from, but since I was 18, I've had a really solid relationship with both of my parents. There are ups and downs to every relationship, but I've gotten a lot closer to each of them. They're a lot happier separate. I'm grateful to have both of them as parents and friends at this point.

You've only got three months of recovery under your belt, what do you think are some of the keys to staying sober?

I know some of the keys for me are keeping open communication lines with my family and the support group that I built. I have a sponsor. I have two service commitments. I live in a sober living environment.

This is my first go-around at recovery. When asked, "What are the keys of success to recovery?" I don't feel like I have those answers. All I know is what's working for me. What's keeping me sober is working an honest program the best that I can. I call my sponsor at least once a week; I text her every day. I sit down and I write every day. I've gotten in contact with my higher power. I turned things over. I surround myself with people who are in recovery who want this. That's just what's worked for me so far.

I personally believe that being in contact with your higher power, whatever that higher power is, is a key part of getting in touch with yourself spiritually and helping yourself to make the right decisions. Could you describe to me what your higher power is?

I don't know exactly what my higher power is, to be honest. Since I've gone in treatment, I've always had this need to put a physical appearance on my higher power. I still struggle with it. To my knowledge, my higher power is the fellowship, the groups, the meetings, everyone who attends, everyone who wants recovery, everyone who is trying at recovery. That's a hard question for me to answer because I can't even formulate that answer in my head. All I know is that there's something out there that is larger than me that will relieve my stress if I turn it over, if I turn my burdens over, if all my insecurities and my weaknesses and my downfalls and all that, I have someone or something to turn it over to. It doesn't even necessarily have to be someone. I have something to turn all of my flaws over to. That's worked for me so far.

In your three months of being clean, how many times have you seriously thought about using cocaine or alcohol?

Every day—that's one of the great things about living at this house, the level of accountability. Also, one of the amazing things about having a really solid group of sober friends is that when I wake up in the morning and I'm like "I really want to go to a bar right now. I want to go sit there and I want to socialize. I want to get drunk," they ground me. They bring me back and they say, "For what reason? What would you get out of that?" Realistically, every day I've thought about picking up, but the level of accountability that I'm holding myself to and the level of accountability that everyone around me is holding me to has kept me sober.

Personally, I found that the first six months of my own recovery from drugs and alcohol, I was telling myself "No" a lot. Thoughts would come into my mind and I'd have to tell myself, "No, don't do that. You can't do that. Stop thinking like that." After six months, it came to me that I was moving toward something new. I was no longer moving away from something. I was now moving toward something new that I wanted, and it was not drugs or alcohol. It was new things in my life that I was trying to move toward, positive things. Have you got any ideas of what you would like to move toward?

I want to go back to school. I want to figure out what I enjoy doing in life. I feel like I really lost that when I started drinking and started not paying attention, especially when I was going to Cabrillo. I had every door open for me that possibly could have been opened, and I took advantage of it and really messed it up. The biggest thing for me is that I feel like I have enough time to figure it out. I don't feel like the anxious pressure of I have to figure it out right this second, but I feel the freedom, and I feel the opportunities that sobriety has brought to me. And I'm grateful for that.

Amanda, you've been wonderful. Thanks for being so honest and so forthright in your answers. I want to give you an opportunity to speak to any suffering addicts who may be considering turning their life around the way that you've managed to turn yours around. It's a fantastic achievement to have three months of sobriety

414

and I wish you 30 years more. What would your message be to the suffering addict?

Thank you. My message would be that every day is not the best day, but every day it gets better. It does. There's not a single day that I don't wake up and feel content with myself because I am not hung over. I wake up every day grateful and ready to start my day and I am excited. I feel the love from my family that I haven't felt in a really long time. I hope that they feel the love from me. I have an amazing community around me of people who I would have never met had I not started on this road. I feel very blessed for every opportunity that I get—not that I get, that I've earned. I have earned the opportunities that are in front of me because I am clean and sober. It gets so much better when you can think clearly. Sobriety really is worth it.

Thank you for that message. And once again, thanks very much for speaking with me.

Epilogue

Does this book inspire you to be part of the solution?

I, Paul Noddings, the author of this book, am reaching out to investors and partners to develop Very High Density Metropolitan Housing, Detox Centers and Purpose Designed Sober Homes.

For many years, I have been a part of the solution to the drug addiction, mental health and homeless crisis in California, using my own capital. I would play a bigger role if I had the support of a philanthropic billionaire or access to significant capital.

If this subject is of interest to you, please contact me for detailed discussions:

Website: www.ResponsibleRecovery.net

Email: info@ResponsibleRecovery.net

Cell Phone: 1-831-818-1186

Made in the USA
Middletown, DE
19 February 2021

33408372R00235